THE SOLAR BODY

TWELVE

ALSO BY ILCHI LEE

THE SOLAR BODY
THE SECRET TO NATURAL HEALING

ILCHI LEE

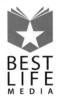

BEST
LIFE
MEDIA

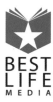

BEST Life Media
6560 State Route 179, Suite 220
Sedona, AZ 86351
www.bestlifemedia.com
877-504-1106

First paperback edition: July 2015
Library of Congress Control Number: 2015934608
ISBN-13: 978-1-935127-75-8

Our original mind is bright like the sun,
and seeks its own brightness.

— *ChunBuKyung (The Heavenly Code), ancient Korean text*

CONTENTS

Chapter 2
The Solar Body Method

Chapter 3

Living as a Solar Body

Chapter 4

Stories of Healing and Empowerment

AUTHOR'S INTRODUCTION

In Sedona, Arizona, where I live, many wildflowers and grasses grow and give off intense life energy under the hot desert sun. Of these, lately I am bewitched by sage. If I put a sage leaf in my mouth and chew it, my body grows warmer and my head clearer. The fragrance and life force of the leaf seem to circulate through my blood vessels, bringing vitality to my whole body. I'm moved by renewed wonder as I vividly feel the changes caused by sage's encounter with my body.

What has given this pungent plant its special qualities? Where did the gentle texture of the sage leaf, the white fuzz covering the back of the leaf, and this refreshing aroma come from?

The power that makes sage into sage is no different from the power that causes the sun to rise and set, the power that makes my heart beat automatically, and the power that causes the salmon to swim upstream, breaking its body on its way to spawn. All these powers ultimately come from the same source.

The breath of the Tao dwelling in perfect form even in a single leaf of sage—this great power and life force of nature—grants sustainability and stability to everything that exists. It is what enables the whole to maintain harmony and balance. When an organism is sick because it has lost its balance, this power is manifest as the natural healing ability that restores balance, returning the organism to a healthy state.

This book contains my proposal for how to use this great restorative power of life—our natural healing ability—to live a healthier, happier, and more meaningful life.

THE GREAT LIFE FORCE WITHIN

We are learning new things every day as we live in a world where we can obtain information more quickly and easily than ever before. The medical arts are gradually developing, and the number of hospitals, doctors, and medicines is increasing. Yet around us, more and more people are sick. Our possessions and knowledge are growing, but we're losing our connection with the great life force that dwells in all things. This life force is the power that makes sage into sage, the power that makes human beings human, and the power that enables each and every one of us to realize our own value and to become who we truly are meant to be.

Losing our connection with this power means losing our connection with ourselves. And as this has happened, we've gradually lost our healthy life rhythm and our self-control. We've come to depend on hospitals and medicines for everything instead of respecting and relying on the natural healing power within us, and working to maintain and recover our own health.

This tendency extends beyond us as individuals to society and the earth as a whole. As our relationship with the life force connecting all things has weakened, our relationship with other people has become superficial. We've come to the point of competing and fighting rather than helping and protecting each other. This goes for our relationship with nature, too. Our natural environment is being destroyed ruthlessly because we've lost much of our ability to sympathize with other life-forms and with the earth itself—the foundation of our lives.

What we can be thankful for is that this life force itself continues to exist perfectly, despite the fact that our connection to it has weakened. Our bodies have a system for providing support, enabling life to maintain itself in optimum condition and to perfectly express its values. If we just avoid getting in the way, good health manifests itself as an obvious and natural phenomenon. A body that has lost balance wants to return to good health, because health is the most natural state of life.

Restoring our connection with the great life force and recovering our natural healing ability doesn't mean simply becoming physically healthier. It means restoring our purest and most natural essence. In the most fundamental sense, it means recovering the true, original nature of humanity. When we are reconnected with this absolute power that brings balance and harmony to all things, we find that our own sense of harmony and balance has been revived within us.

I believe the key to solving everything from individual problems to the global environmental crisis or political and religious conflicts is to be found in restoring this link with the great life force. By recovering our natural healing ability and the goodness of human nature, we can create a truly peaceful, sustainable world.

And I don't believe that these are things that social institutions or prestigious experts can do for us: they must happen within each and every one of us.

THE SOLAR BODY CONCEPT

In this book, I am presenting the new concept of the Solar Body. What do I mean by this? "Solar Body" refers to someone who creates her own health and happiness by recovering her natural healing power, making herself shine brightly like the sun.

It doesn't take complex technology or tremendous effort to recover natural healing power and achieve a Solar Body. The Solar Body isn't about creating an amazingly muscular physique, or developing an enviably slender waistline. It's about reviving a sense for the balance and harmony that exist perfectly within us.

The secret of natural healing power—the heart of the Solar Body concept—is found in a linking of three elements: body temperature, breathing, and the power of the observing mind. When, by concentrating our minds, we feel our body heat and observe our breathing, we recover the desired balance of body temperature, with the head cool and the lower abdomen warm. Breathing naturally grows deeper and slower. The life energy in our bodies is activated and circulates, and our natural healing power manifests best in this state.

In this book, I introduce some simple but powerful methods of meditation and exercise for maximizing natural healing power. The Solar Body Method is made up of Sunlight Meditation, to receive solar energy directly from sunlight; Solar Energy Circuit

Training, for total transformative healing with focused awareness; and Solar Body Exercises, for increasing body temperature and recovering optimal energy balance through movement.

Throughout my life, I have researched methods for recovering health of body and mind and for developing the potential of the brain, and I've shared what I've learned with many people. Hundreds of thousands of people worldwide have found certain exercises to be effective. Three of the simplest yet most effective—those that best incorporate the principles involved in recovering natural healing power—have been selected for the Solar Body Method. These meditations and exercises look so easy that you might be tempted to question how they could be considered exercise at all. But you'll be surprised by the powerful results.

RECHARGE YOURSELF WITH SOLAR ENERGY

Make the Solar Body Method a part of your life for a time, and your ability to focus on your body—and more fundamentally on yourself—will grow. As your consciousness turns inward, your lost sense of balance and self-control will be revived and your power to examine your own thoughts, emotions, and habits will improve. When your communication with yourself deepens in this way and you develop the power to observe and choose, you will have the power to create positive change—not only in your health but in all areas of your life, including relationships and self-development.

The Solar Body Method is so simple and natural that anyone

can experience its effects and share it with others. And when many people are able to maintain their health with an easy, natural method, medical expenses will be reduced for society as a whole and the quality of life will be improved. The stress we put on nature will also be reduced. Each of us recovering our own healing abilities, and helping others to do the same, will bring gentle yet powerful and fundamental changes to human life. That in turn will create a peaceful and sustainable world, in effect increasing the natural healing power of the planet itself.

What's important is that these changes can begin with very small things. I recommend that you start by trying the Solar Body Method for just one week. Set aside about 30 minutes a day to do the three exercises. You'll be surprised by the many positive changes such simple-seeming exercises will create in your body and mind. I can say this with confidence, for I've experienced it myself. And over the past 30 years, countless people around the world have experienced fundamental life changes this way.

Now it's your turn. Through the Solar Body Method, may you awaken the infinite life force latent in your body and mind. May you live a fantastic life overflowing with vitality, passion, and significance. I hope that, through this book, you will be able to experience with your whole body the simple yet powerful truth that your health, happiness, and peace are truly up to you.

Ilchi Lee
Spring 2015 in Sedona

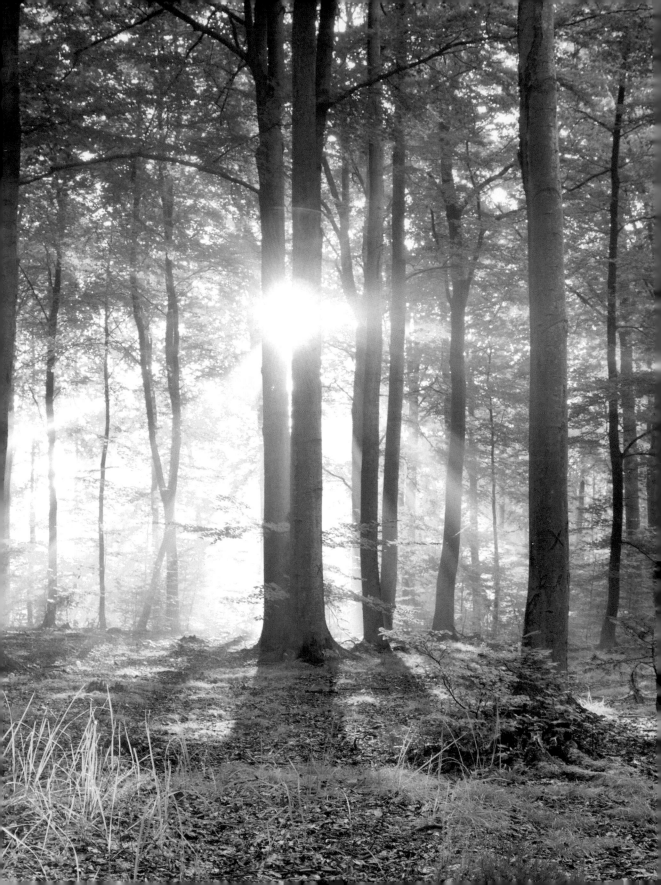

CHAPTER 1

RECOVERING YOUR **NATURAL** HEALING POWER

HEALTH IS
NOT A LUXURY

BECOMING HEALTHY NATURALLY

Traveling around the world and lecturing on the mind–body training methods I've developed, I have met many people who are ailing in body and mind. I have also seen many people who have been healed miraculously after suffering with long illnesses and mental pain. In this process, I became painfully aware that physical and mental health are an important foundation for quality of life. Many other good things in life pale in significance if you lose your health.

With the development of science, technology, and modern medicine, our lives have truly become more convenient, and our average lifespan has increased. However, our health and happiness don't seem to have increased much. The number of hospitals and doctors increases, and new medicines are constantly being developed and advertised. Why, then, do we find ourselves surrounded by a growing number of sick people?

According to the statistics, 70 percent of Americans say they're taking medication for some health problem. To put it another way, 70 percent of them are sick. Medical costs amount to 17 percent of the country's gross domestic product, and medical expenditures account for the largest percentage of government expenditures—at 28 percent, more than defense spending. Comparing annual per capita medical costs with those of other countries that have a similar standard of living, the United States has virtually the worst score in various major health indices—including infant mortality, average lifespan, obesity rates, and cancer rates—even while spending close to three times as much as the average. (This information was gathered from member nations of the Organization for Economic Co-operation and Development, or OECD.) It appears to have a very inefficient system in terms of cost-effectiveness, and as a result the burden of family medical expenses is one of the most significant causes of personal bankruptcy.

Two major indices highlighting this inefficiency are per capita drug consumption and the number of high-tech diagnostic devices mobilized for medical treatment. Approximately $600 billion worth of medications are consumed worldwide each year. Half of that, $300 billion worth, is consumed in the United States. Yet the U.S. population, at about 320 million, accounts for no more than 5 percent of global population. Less than 5 percent of the world's population accounts for 50 percent of global drug consumption! As for diagnostic devices, the OECD average for the use of MRI machines is 13 units per million people. The United States uses 37 units per million—almost three times the average.

Excessive use of medicines and equipment is a significant cause of the country's high-cost health-care structure. An uncomfortable truth is that overprescription of drugs and overuse of high-tech diagnostic equipment is for the benefit of the pharmaceutical industry rather than the patient, and for the industry to protect itself from liability-related litigation.

What's important is not simply the cost structure, but whether the system is operating properly, and whether there are alternatives to this approach. Even high costs can be justified if they're effective, because health is very important. If, however, the current high-cost, high-energy medical system is failing to perform its role in improving overall health—and if there are easier, more natural, less expensive ways to obtain and maintain health—then we should really rethink the system.

People who are sick, full of fear, and in despair are all around us. These conditions are closely related. The thought that you might not have money for treatment when you're sick is certainly a cause for fear. Believing that such conditions are not likely to change much in the future leads to despair.

Even though our overall standard of living has greatly improved over the last century, it's an unfortunate irony that we find more sick people around us, and that we're worrying more about health. But the news isn't all bad. The good news is that more of us have started to take serious, fundamental interest in our health. We've started to question the means of maintaining and managing our individual health. We're beginning to ask, "Is this actually the best approach?" And we're starting to actively search for alternatives.

Even better news is the fact that we can recover and maintain health by using a simple, natural approach. It's not about eating or drinking something special, having some special procedure performed, or going to some specific location. Hidden in movements we're always doing—breathing, walking, even shaking and patting ourselves—is the key to making us healthy and vigorous. The secret is hidden in natural phenomena we encounter every day, like solar energy. My goal in writing this book is to place in your hands this key hidden in your own body.

OUR BODIES WANT HEALTH

Things are highly specialized and compartmentalized in today's world, and health is no exception. Many people think they can't take care of their own health without the latest technology or groundbreaking drug. When they develop health problems, they search for treatment methods outside themselves.

Many people believe without question that specialized medical equipment is required to properly analyze and diagnose their physical condition, and even to provide treatment. Depending on complicated, high-tech equipment, we've gradually grown distant from the subtle senses of our bodies, and we've forgotten how great our bodies' self-awareness is.

So many people treat their own bodies like strangers. Having become insensitive to signals from their bodies and having lost self-control, they don't necessarily seek to change. They may know their health is being ruined by their lifestyle choices, but they rely on hospitals and medications when their health has deteriorated irreversibly. The result? Health has become a product we must buy at very high cost from highly trained specialists. We accept this as natural and don't even question it much.

Do we really have to obtain health through specialists alone, and at such a high price? If we'd look around a bit, we'd see that this situation isn't found in other organisms. How many doctors does a mountainside tree have, and what hospitals does an ocean fish visit? Are wild organisms stronger than we are, even though no one cares for them?

What the rest of the natural world shows us is that our bodies are already equipped with a support system for maintaining us in an optimal state. Health occurs as an obvious, natural thing when that system is working well. Health is the most natural state of life. Bodies that have lost their balance want to return to a healthy state.

When a situation is serious and we need the help of medical experts, obviously we should get it. The problem is our overly dependent attitude, our seeking to solve all our problems through an external expert. Our bodies are designed to ceaselessly return to balance and health. That's why anyone can enjoy optimum health through his or her own efforts. We need to take serious interest in our bodies and listen to the signals they send us. We should understand deeply that our bodies want health and have the power to maintain their own health, and we should live our lives in a way that adapts to and strengthens that power.

RETHINKING NATURAL HEALING POWER

YOUR BODY HAS AMAZING ABILITY TO RECOVER BALANCE

If your skin is pierced by a thorn or cut by a sharp object, in time the wound heals and new skin appears. If you get sick from eating bad food, after a painful time of abdominal pain, vomiting, and diarrhea, you'll be able to eat food again. We all experience this kind of healing.

This extends beyond such ordinary cases. We hear stories about how someone with a hard-to-treat disease such as cancer has been healed after completely changing his attitude or lifestyle. Such things are possible because our bodies have an ability to heal themselves; in other words, they have natural healing power. Within our bodies are mechanisms for self-diagnosis, self-restoration, and regeneration. These mechanisms are always ready to go to work restoring balance when it has been broken.

This natural healing power is the ultimate reason why any disease heals, with or without medical intervention such as drugs or surgery. Medical treatments are effective thanks to the operation of this natural internal healing mechanism.

Colds are the most common example of natural healing. These days, people get injections and prescription drugs even for colds. But that doesn't, in fact, cure a cold. Colds are caused by viruses, and there's still no medication that eliminates cold viruses. Fever-reducing and cough-suppressing agents merely alleviate cold symptoms.

The fever, coughing, and runny nose that you get when you have a cold are part of the process of natural healing. Fever is a sign that your immune system has kicked into gear, while the coughing and runny nose are how your body expels secretions that result from inflammation. Medications can suppress the symptoms, but they cannot cure the common cold. What ultimately cures a cold is natural healing power.

Your body really shows its natural healing power if you cut your finger. Your body feels pain and stops the flow of blood within a few minutes, thanks to the action of blood platelets. An inflammatory reaction develops within 24 hours—an immune response created so that white blood cells can stop the invasion of bacteria at the injury site and clear away dead or dying cells. Next, new skin and new blood vessels develop.

The same kind of thing happens when you break one of your bones, the most solid tissue in your body. A simple fracture will heal completely within a few months on its own. Bone cells regenerate at the break site and come together so exquisitely that the fracture no longer shows up on an X-ray in many cases.

Even more impressive is the liver's ability to regenerate lost tissue. Even if you cut out most of the liver (amazingly, up to 80 percent), if the remaining tissue is normal, the lost portions will be restored within hours.

Our bodies are ceaselessly shedding their outermost layer of skin and creating new skin immediately below it. The inner wall of the intestines is also peeled away and replaced every three to six days. The body's regenerative ability is amazing.

Inside and outside us are countless factors causing our body systems—from cells to organs—to move out of a healthy state of balance. Pollutants in the air and water, chemicals and heavy metals in our food, high-frequency electromagnetic waves generated by all sorts of electronic devices, radiation, ultraviolet rays pouring down from the sun—we're constantly being exposed to hazards. These all have an impact on the sensitive and delicate process of cellular replication.

Our bodies are made up of approximately 37 trillion cells. Millions of cells die or are born each second. If carcinogens make something go wrong in even one of the genetic replication processes taking place every time this happens, abnormal cells may develop. Left alone, they could create deformities or grow into tumors, as in cancer.

Cancer is often considered the most difficult disease to treat, but at the same time it is the malady that best demonstrates the body's natural healing abilities. Even in healthy people, abnormal and potentially cancerous cells appear and disappear every day. Millions of these abnormal cells don't develop into cancer, because they're detected and eliminated by the body's internal quarantine function. The very fact that most of us don't get cancer, even though there's so much potential for that to happen, shows the presence of a powerful natural healing ability.

One thing is often misunderstood about cancer: people think cancer cells are vital and tough. In fact, they're the opposite. Cancer cells are much weaker than ordinary cells when it comes to thermal changes, and they also have problems with changes in pH. Ordinary cells can take temperatures up to about 107.6 degrees F (42 degrees C), but cancer cells start to be destroyed at just 100.4°F (38°C). Healthy cells are weakly alkaline, but cancer cells grow well in an acidic environment and can't endure a pH of 7.5 or greater. Physically and chemically, cancer cells are weaker than ordinary cells.

The fundamental reason why cancer treatment is difficult is not that cancerous cells are strong, but that the body's internal self-correction system has been broken. In other words, its natural healing ability is weakened. The very fact that cancer cells have developed means that the body's function for detecting and removing these cells isn't operating normally. That's why it's not realistic to expect a fundamental cure for cancer without strengthening the body's natural healing power.

The vital phenomena arising in our bodies, including natural healing, can only be described as marvelous. Cells numbering more than 5,000 times the globe's human population spontaneously achieve harmony, make up for inadequacies, and reduce excesses to find perfect balance. Compared with the natural healing that takes place automatically within each of us, our efforts to consciously promote our own health are really quite trivial.

WHAT'S THE SOURCE OF OUR NATURAL HEALING POWER?

When the balance in our bodies is broken, where does the tendency and power to restore that original balance—this amazing, even mysterious natural healing ability—come from? I believe that it comes from a place much more fundamental than cells or DNA.

According to modern physics, everything in existence has the basic properties of variability and uncertainty. Large things are made up of small things. Elementary particles come together to form atoms, atoms come together to form molecules, and they also come together to form the cells that make up our organs and bodies. The whole is variable and uncertain, beginning with these smallest components. The universe, our bodies, even immeasurably small elementary particles—all are variable and uncertain.

If everything is so variable and uncertain, how then do our bodies maintain a sustainable, stable state? It's not simply our bodies, either. This is the way of all organisms—and of the earth, the solar system, and, moreover, the entire universe.

There are many physical forces at work to achieve this homeostatic harmony. For it to be maintained, energy needs to be constantly put in. Without it, particles could not even come together in the first place, and systems of all sizes would fall apart.

However, how did it all start and why? What keeps the system going despite the natural tendency toward variability and chaos? It seems as if some benevolent mind that earnestly longs to create something from nothing, harmony out of chaos, willed it into being. As a result, all life exists and has an opportunity to realize its potential value and to create new possibilities.

Natural healing power is normally considered the same as immunity, but the source of our healing ability exists in a much deeper place. The power of the universal mind that bestows sustainability and stability on all things, that enables the whole to maintain harmony and balance—that is the source of natural healing ability. The same power that enables healing to occur automatically in my body isn't separate from the power behind the force that keeps the earth on its path orbiting the sun, the force that makes water flow downhill, or the drive of the salmon to swim upstream to spawn. It's the power behind the instinct that sends a baby kangaroo, smaller than your finger, crawling with eyes closed far up its mother's belly into the pouch containing milk. It's the power ensuring that everything maintains balance, order, and harmony even within dynamic movement—the force that provides sustainability and stability even within the potential for infinite change. That force penetrates and connects all things, from single particles to the entire universe.

Recovering natural healing ability doesn't simply signify becoming physically healthier. It means recovering our sense of the natural, pure essence that animates us. It means rediscovering from that sense the judgment to make good choices—choices beneficial to oneself and to the whole—without even thinking about it. More fundamentally, it means coming to realize what I really am. Within the ceaseless, coming-and-going change and uncertainty, I discover the essence of my dauntlessly existing, eternal self.

This realization revives our sense of connection with everything around us, our sense of harmony with the whole. It gives us the wisdom to see through to the essence of things and to solve problems. This gives us the power to choose and create, and the internal peace and courage not to be shaken by the environment surrounding us. In its most fundamental sense, this is about rediscovering the "humanness" of humanity—the true, original nature of humans.

TURN ON YOUR HEALING MODE

WHAT PUTS THE BRAKES ON NATURAL HEALING POWER?

Why are so many people around us hurting if everyone has natural healing power? Physical abnormalities that are temporary and not serious, like colds or light injuries, are a natural part of human life. However, far too many people suffer from diseases that, due to their chronic nature and severity, are a significant hindrance to living high-quality lives. Unfortunately, the number of such people continues to grow.

If we're suffering from chronic diseases because the natural healing power of our bodies isn't operating as it should, ruining our mechanisms for self-diagnosis, self-restoration, and self-regeneration, what is it that's keeping it from working? What can we do to release our healing power and recover health and vitality?

Stress is said to be the source of innumerable diseases. It has a huge impact on natural healing power, too. Chronic stress is the most powerful brake keeping natural healing power from manifesting itself.

The body's stress reaction is regulated by the autonomic nervous system. This system is connected from the brain through the spinal cord to all the major organs in our bodies. All vital functions —breathing, sleeping, digestion, the beating of the heart, the rise and fall of body temperature—are regulated and managed by the autonomic nervous system, which helps our bodies maintain equilibrium. The autonomic nervous system is the key to stability and balance in our bodies.

The survival instinct is one of the toughest programs installed in living things. Survival means not dying by accident or disease— the two greatest threats to life. Although these are both threats, they require different modes of response. Not dying by accident requires a quick and effective emergency response to unanticipated threats. To avoid dying from disease, vital functions must be maintained to facilitate resistance to pathogens and a constant, sustained response to pathogens is needed.

The body's autonomic nervous system has two subsystems, antagonistic in character and complementary in function, for dealing effectively with these two dangers. One is the *sympathetic nervous system*, the other the *parasympathetic nervous system*. The sympathetic subsystem handles emergency response to unforeseen dangers, helping us escape death by accident. The parasympathetic subsystem handles rest, recharging, and healing, helping us avoid death from disease. The sympathetic nervous system excites us, allowing us to deal with danger through the fight-or-flight response. On the other hand, the parasympathetic nervous system relaxes us. It replenishes our energy through digestion, handles excretion of toxins, and repairs injuries.

Our bodies can safely maintain vital activity over the long term through the cooperation and balance of these two systems. Their cooperative relationship shows a perfect harmony that operates in humans today just the same as it did in our ancestors millions of years ago.

The reason more people seem to be getting sick and suffering from chronic illnesses these days isn't that their autonomic nervous systems have been weakened or broken, but that they continue to operate perfectly. A little more concretely, today's lifestyles involving sustained stress simply don't mesh well with the normal mode of cooperation between the sympathetic and parasympathetic nervous systems.

These two subsystems have a kind of seesaw relationship, interacting and maintaining balance: when one side grows stronger the other grows weaker. When we perceive a situation as a crisis, causing stress, the sympathetic nervous system takes the initiative and controls our bodies and brains. Meanwhile, functions controlled by the parasympathetic nervous system are weakened or temporarily suspended. Since we have to respond to an immediate crisis, functions that can be performed when the situation is less pressing—digestion, detoxification, and healing—are temporarily shut down. After all, digestion, healing, and rest are meaningless unless we survive the immediate crisis.

When our sympathetic nervous system is excited by a crisis situation, a chain of stress reactions is instantly triggered. Blood drains from the internal organs (including the digestive system) and concentrates in the large muscles of the arms and legs, a condition favorable for fight or flight. The activity of the cerebral cortex—involved in thinking, analysis-synthesis, and judgment—comes to a stop. Glucose is secreted from the liver to supply the muscles with energy, raising blood sugar levels and making the blood thick and sticky, which facilitates coagulation. The heartbeat speeds up and blood pressure increases for a rapid supply of blood. To put it another way, conditions of hypertension, diabetes, heart disease, arteriosclerosis, perceptual disorder, and indigestion are temporarily created. Incredible potential energy is generated in the body to make possible the explosive action necessary for responding to a crisis. But unless this energy is discharged through action, its destructive force is turned inward, damaging cells, tissues, and organs.

This isn't ordinarily a problem for animals in nature. Such a hyper-activated state lasts no more than about three minutes for an impala being chased by a lioness in search of food for its family. Live or die, the impala will have its fate decided within three minutes because a lion can't run at top speed for longer than that. If the impala runs faster than the lion for three minutes or more, the threat to its survival ends and sympathetic dominance changes to parasympathetic dominance. The impala's physiological functions are safely protected, because the explosive energy created by this stress reaction was fully released during its brief flight for life.

In this way, parasympathetic dominance normally is maintained most of the time for healthy organisms in their natural state. They enter a state of sympathetic dominance temporarily only when it's necessitated by an emergency. The situation is different for people, however. Why? We restlessly create stress through the power of our mental capabilities—memory, thought, imagination—even when no physical threat exists. Thus the light of our sympathetic nervous system is always turned on, ready to deal with crisis situations, and our parasympathetic nervous system continues to be suppressed.

If this continues for long, our bodies don't have time to replenish energy, eliminate toxins, and repair damage. The explosive energy generated through the stress reaction turns inward, damaging cells, tissues, and organs. Meanwhile, the inability to continue supplying the kind of energy required by the stress reaction results in depleted energy; fatigued nerves, organs, and muscles; and reduced blood circulation. Problems develop in the autonomic nervous system, resulting in weakened immunity and chaotic endocrine function. The key to good health—balance—is broken, and the body loses its regulatory ability.

It's like stepping on the accelerator with one foot while pressing on the brake with the other, and continuing to drive that way without maintaining your car. The power created by the engine is being used to damage the car and not actually to move it. The damage continues, appropriate maintenance isn't done, and nuts and bolts may start to fall out. Then rattles develop, oil and cooling fluids leak, belts break, and eventually the car is no longer drivable. In our bodies, this shows up as disease.

The stress reaction is essential for protecting the body when it faces an outside threat. But problems occur if that condition continues too long. There's a good reason why stress is called the root of all illness. Suppressing the parasympathetic system—which plays the most important role in the body's natural healing ability—makes it impossible for the entire autonomic nervous system to operate in a balanced way. In this sense, an important element in helping our bodies to express their natural healing power is shutting down the emergency-response system and turning on parasympathetic pre-dominance. That's when rest, replenishing, and healing take place.

THREE SWITCHES FOR TURNING ON THE HEALING MODE

How can we switch our bodies from chronic stress mode to healing mode? What is an effective way to switch from a mode of tension and emergency response to a mode of rest, recharging, and healing?

Many approaches are used to alleviate stress, from reaching for something to eat or drink to exercise, deep breathing, meditation, and even autosuggestion and positive thinking. In this book, I am introducing a method of restoring natural healing power that has these important conditions: it should be able to be done by yourself without external help, and it has to be a natural approach, not an artificial one. Based on these conditions, I propose three switches for turning on your healing mode:

- First, feel your body heat.
- Second, control your breathing.
- Third, observe with your mind.

What's important here is using these three things simultaneously. Body temperature, respiration, and observation with the mind—each is an effective tool for managing stress and restoring natural healing power. Their effects are maximized to an amazing degree, though, when they are used together.

Body temperature and breathing are especially important—not only because they are simple tools for managing stress, but because they are the most central elements of natural healing ability. I'll discuss this in detail in the next section, but temperature is one of the physical conditions that exerts the most direct influence on our bodies, including the immune system and metabolic rate. And our breathing both influences and directly reflects the balance of the autonomic nervous system. It can be a powerful tool for strengthening natural healing ability, restoring balance in the autonomic nervous system, and regulating the stress reaction.

By peacefully observing its own thoughts and emotions, the mind has the power to restore balance to the elements of the body's natural healing ability. Your busy mind will grow quiet and find composure when you concentrate on the here and now and feel your breathing and body temperature.

FEEL YOUR BODY HEAT

WHY IS BODY TEMPERATURE IMPORTANT?

We usually don't think about our body temperature unless we're very hot or cold. We don't necessarily need to—it's regulated automatically, just like our heartbeat and breathing. Beginning now, though, I want you to take an active interest. Body temperature has an immense impact on your health and happiness, for body temperature contains an important secret to recovering natural healing power.

The most important of the internal conditions required to maintain life are called our "vital signs." These are our heart rate (pulse), blood pressure, body temperature, and respiration rate. Which of these has the narrowest range for what's considered normal? Body temperature.

A normal heart rate at rest is about 70 beats per minute. Individual differences are large, though, so 60 to 100 is considered normal. There's also a large difference between one's maximum and minimum heart rate under normal conditions, about 100 beats per minute. The greater this difference, the stronger a person's resistance to stress and the healthier they're considered.

The range for normal blood pressure is also large—90 to 120 millimeters Hg for systolic pressure, 60 to 80 mm Hg for diastolic.

Compared with heart rate and blood pressure, the normal range for body temperature is extremely narrow, between 97.7 and 99.5 degrees F (36.5–37.5 degrees C). One's life is at risk if body temperature drops 3.6–5.4 degrees F or rises 7.2–9.0 degrees F.

Metabolism—the rate at which your body converts food into energy—is reduced approximately 12 percent when body temperature drops by just 1.8 degrees F. Shivering is the first reaction when temperature starts to drop. The body's temperature-regulating system makes the muscles shake in order to raise the temperature. As temperature continues to fall, movement becomes sluggish. Hand movement becomes unnatural, gait becomes shaky, and symptoms of slight delirium are seen. Peripheral blood vessels contract to preserve heat, causing blood pressure to rise, and the heart beats faster to make up for heat loss. Even a healthy person can die of a heart attack in this condition, because the heart goes into overdrive to raise body temperature.

Fever above the normal range is also risky. What is impacted first and most fatally is brain function. Headache develops, hallucinations occur, and heatstroke can occur.

What has been revealed through many clinical studies is that body temperature is deeply related to the immune system. Immunity increases when body temperature rises within the normal range and decreases when it falls. If pathogens such as bacteria or viruses invade the body, the immune system increases body temperature while it fights them. Temperature returns to normal when symptoms are alleviated.

What do we need most to maintain life? Food to eat and air to breathe probably come to mind first. But the reason we eat food is to burn it for energy, and we breathe in oxygen to burn that food and change it into energy. Put another way, rather than being essential in themselves, food and breathing are needed in the process of metabolism for obtaining energy through combustion. And we don't only obtain energy in this process. As when we burn fuel in an automobile, waste products remain after combustion. If these accumulate, they bring disease and accelerate aging. Ultimately, the very functions of life stop. If we could obtain energy without going through this process of chemical conversion, it would be groundbreaking for preventing aging and extending life.

What we should understand here is that it's not food or breathing that life ultimately needs, but energy. And the most direct expression of energy is heat. In this sense, temperature expresses the essence of life. When you feel the heat in your body, you're observing the most central operations of your life. You're connected to the essence of life.

Temperature doesn't affect only our bodies. Temperature is powerful enough to determine whether or not all organisms on our planet survive. If the earth were just a little closer to the sun or a little farther away, the change in temperature would make impossible the creation of a biosphere like the one we have now. Our current ecosystem is sustained because the planet maintains a temperature suitable for biological activity. If a collision with an asteroid or a volcanic explosion were to obscure the sun's light, the planet's existing flora and fauna would disappear, unable to last even a month without heat and light.

The rising sea level and ecosystem changes caused by global warming create the biggest environmental crisis humanity now faces. Some may think that the whole earth will become like a sauna if global warming proceeds, but in fact it's a temperature change of just a few degrees that is bringing this great crisis.

Temperature is an absolute and essential condition for maintaining life on earth, and at the same time it's the most subtle and sensitive one. That is why I consider body temperature the most important key to recovering natural healing power. If we really understand and utilize temperature, we'll be able to live lives overflowing with health and vitality by creating in our bodies a climate capable of maximizing our healing power.

INCREASE YOUR BODY TEMPERATURE AT LEAST ONCE A DAY

All organisms have their own vital temperature necessary for maintaining a healthy life. Their life force declines and they readily become sick unless they maintain this unique temperature.

The normal temperature of the human body is 97.7–99.5 degrees F. Although body temperature changes constantly depending on the environment, the weather, and the time of day as well as the condition of the body and mind, being outside this range for long brings many health problems.

Many people are in a continuous state of low body temperature. Try taking your temperature a couple of hours after you get up in the morning. If it measures lower than 97.7°F you're considered to be verging on hypothermic. There's a close connection between low body temperature and many diseases that modern people experience. Most people who are obese, have a chronic disease such as diabetes or hypertension, or suffer from depression have a lower-than-average body temperature.

Experts researching the correlation between health and body temperature say that maintaining a temperature close to 98.6°F—in other words, just a little high within the normal range—is an effective way to increase natural healing ability and maintain physical and mental health and vitality.

Falling body temperature weakens blood circulation, metabolism, and detoxification. Blood vessels contract when the body becomes colder, inhibiting circulation. And since blood transports the nutrients, oxygen, and moisture that the body requires, when it doesn't flow smoothly the organs don't receive what they need for their activity. As metabolism declines, unused energy accumulates, even leading to obesity. Ambition and passion for life fade.

Blood also transports waste products generated in the body. If the body gets colder and blood circulation problems develop, these waste products accumulate. This can cause contamination and a decline in cell function, often leading to disease.

Yet another problem is that white blood cell activity decreases when body temperature drops. We depend on our white blood cells, or leukocytes, to dismantle invading bacteria and build our immune system, fighting viruses, parasites, mold, pollen, and other pathogens. White blood cells also protect the body by attacking tumors, preventing the creation of cancer cells, and eliminating virus-infected cells before they can damage other cells. But when low body temperature weakens the immune system, this defense system collapses.

Elevated body temperature, on the other hand, is known to increase the activity of immune-function cells, and to boost energy production by elevating the metabolic rate. We know that cold-blooded animals lower their body temperature and their metabolic rate to make it through the winter when there's nothing to eat. According to Japanese immunologist Dr. Toru Abo of Niigata University, the immune system is strengthened fivefold when body temperature increases just 1.8 degrees F (1 degree C). Conversely, it's weakened by 35 percent when body temperature drops this same amount.

Heat therapies, in fact, have been in use for a very long time. In the East, moxibustion has been an important treatment for several millennia. It involves thermal stimulation from medicinal herbs burned on specific parts of the body. There are records indicating that Hippocrates, born nearly 2,500 years ago and known as the "father of medicine," used heat to treat patients.

Many things can cause body temperature to fall. Chronic stress can lead to a decline in the functioning of the autonomic nervous system and peripheral circulatory disorders, resulting in colder extremities and lower body temperature. Decrease in muscle mass can cause low body temperature. Muscles are our greatest organ for generating heat—the boilers of our bodies. About 25 percent of the heat generated in the body is created in the muscles. More than 70 percent of our muscles are in the lower body, and if we're lazy about exercising them it's easy for the body to get cold.

Overeating, cold food, excessive air conditioning, inadequate sleep, and frequent use of fever reducers and pain relievers—all of these things can make the body cold. If we overeat, blood gathers in the stomach to digest the food. Bodily movement decreases and temperature falls because less blood then goes to the brain, hands, feet, and muscles.

Develop a habit of keeping your body warm in your daily life, and try to increase your body temperature by just one or two degrees at least once or twice a day by using the Solar Body Method. Improving your blood and energy circulation by raising your temperature through exercise and meditation, and not from being sick, will give you the gift of health and vitality. You'll be amazed at how great the slight change of body temperature you create for yourself will make you feel, both in body and in mind.

HEAD COOL, BELLY WARM

Even if your body temperature measures a certain number of degrees on a thermometer, the whole body is almost never uniformly that temperature. Some parts are warmer than others. The question is, which parts are cooler and which ones warmer? Ordinarily, the closer you get to the core of the body, the higher the temperature; the farther away from the core, the lower the temperature. What's particularly important is the temperature balance between the head and the abdomen.

Which should be cool and which should be warm? We can know intuitively that the head should be cool and the belly warm. But this balance is reversed when we're under stress or we catch a cold. Then our heads get hot and our bellies cold. We feel frustrated and dazed, and struggle to think clearly. Our internal organs are unable to move smoothly, causing our metabolism to drop, preventing excretion of toxins, and resulting in indigestion or constipation.

It may seem strange in the Western world, but in the East this has been known for millennia as a basic principle of good health. It's called Water-up, Fire-down. Occurring automatically in a healthy organism, this balance has become more and more difficult to maintain in modern times as chronic stress has increased. Thus it has become that much more important.

As we hear in common, everyday language, we know intuitively that the brain should be cool and the abdomen warm—and that stress usually reverses this. "That person is such a hothead!" we say to describe someone who's upset or stressed out, or "He's hot under the collar." On the other hand, you've also heard people say, "She keeps her cool," "Cool heads prevail," or "I'm going to go blow off some steam."

Water-up, Fire-down is an optimal energy state that facilitates the function of all the organs and maximizes brain vitality. When you achieve Water-up, Fire-down, not only do you overflow with energy and vitality, but level-headed judgment and wisdom emerge within you. Your mind becomes stable and more peaceful.

In contrast, if your temperature balance reversed so that fire energy collects in your head, then your natural healing power is weakened. Your mouth becomes dry and bitter as your brain grows hot and your belly cold, and your heart beats irregularly. You're tired and anxious, you have malaise, and your neck and shoulders feel stiff. Most people experience digestive dysfunction when water energy rather than fire energy accumulates in the lower abdomen. Their intestines stiffen, their lower abdomen becomes hard and painful to the touch, and constipation develops. They may develop cold extremities.

What keeps us from achieving Water-up, Fire-down? The most significant reason is stress. Your neck is where you first start tensing when you're under stress, particularly where your skull and spine meet at the first cervical vertebra. When this spot is stiff, tension spreads through your shoulders and back to your entire spine. Neck stiffness inhibits the blood flow rising along your neck to your head, preventing a smooth supply to your brain. At the same time, tension in your chest suppresses natural breathing, interrupting the gas exchange in your lungs. Blood circulation to the brain is inhibited, and the blood that is supplied doesn't contain enough oxygen. It becomes difficult for the brain to operate normally, causing heat to build up and producing a "hot head." That can lead to migraine headaches, hypertension, stroke, and other nervous system disorders.

Imbalance caused by chronic stress can be considered the prevalent condition of modern people in regard to body temperature. If we correct this imbalance—keeping our bodies warm overall while our heads stay cooler and our lower abdomens warmer—natural healing ability will be restored. Good health will follow.

RAISE THE TEMPERATURE
OF YOUR MIND

Not long ago, I came across a fascinating research report show-ing that sensory temperature changes follow emotional changes. These experimental results were published in January 2014 in the *Proceedings of the National Academy of Sciences of the United States of America (PNAS)* in the article "Body maps of emotions" by Lauri Nummenmaaa, et al.

A research team at Aalto University in Finland conducted a study on about 700 subjects in three countries: Sweden, Finland, and Taiwan. The subjects colored silhouettes of bodies to indicate where in their own bodies they felt temperature changes and other physical changes when they experienced particular emo-tions while looking at different words or images. On one silhouette they colored in areas where they felt more bodily sensations and on another silhouette they colored areas where they felt less. Test results indicated that subjects who experienced anger or fear felt greater sensation in their chests. Those who felt sadness or depres-sion felt their arms and legs more. Participants who felt happy had greater sensation spreading evenly throughout their bodies, not just in specific areas. Those who felt the emotion of love felt more sensation over their upper bodies, but not their lower bodies.

The study didn't use objective equipment, but instead recorded the subjective feelings of test participants. However, subjects exhibited common reactions, regardless of differences in culture or gender, showing that people can feel and be aware of general physiological changes, such as temperature, in the body.

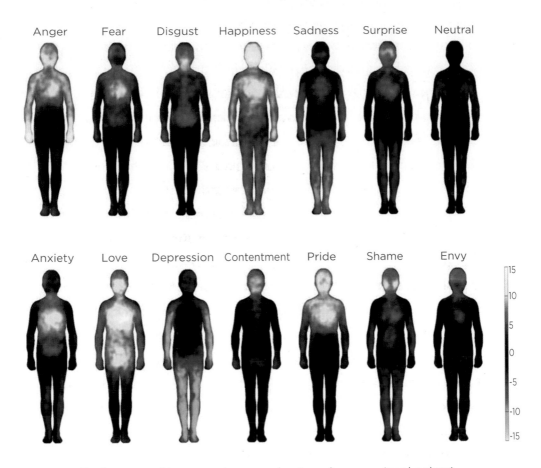

Body maps of increase (warm colors) or decrease (cool colors) in subjective physical sensations of emotions.

This connection doesn't exist only at the level of subjective perception. Body temperature changes according to our surrounding environment or physical and physiological activity, but it also changes according to our emotional state. Emotions bring physiological changes through our body's hormonal systems, and these lead to changes in body temperature. When you're afraid, excited, or angry, your body temperature changes accordingly. If you are mired in an unhealthy emotional state such as worry, anxiety, anger, or sadness, you become depressed and everything becomes irritating. You don't even want to move. Your body temperature drops naturally when you're in this condition.

Our body temperature reaches about 97.7 degrees F (36.5°C) when we're in a comfortable state of rest or when we're meditating, and it reaches about 99.5°F (37.5°C) when we are most active, physically and mentally. That's why I call 97.7°F the "temperature of recovery" and 99.5°F the "temperature of passion."

When the mind is healthy, our body's temperature is in a healthy state. But when the mind experiences an emotional roller coaster or depression, our body temperature moves out of the normal range. That's why it's important to be diligent about managing our minds if we are to maintain a healthy body temperature—to think positively and to have a passionate attitude toward life. Just as you aim to raise your body temperature slightly through exercise and meditation at least once a day, look into your heart and mind and fill yourself with passion for life and hope at least once each day.

The advantage of the Solar Body Method is that it allows you to raise the temperature of your body and the temperature of your mind together. It begins in "feeling" your body heat. You can't feel your body heat unless your mind focuses on your body. When you feel your body by directing your awareness inward, your body will grow warmer, its energy circulation will be activated, and your once-roiling emotions, stress, and outward-directed thoughts will quiet down. Your body's natural healing power will improve, and you'll have renewed passion.

CONTROL YOUR BREATHING

THE POWER OF BREATHING

Try to hold your breath right now for about a minute. How does it feel? In no time at all, your chest feels tight, your blood pressure rises, and your head starts hurting. Now exhale the breath you've been holding. Your chest will feel relieved, your head refreshed, and your body relaxed. In just this way, breathing directly impacts the health of our bodies and minds. It's no great threat to life to go without food or water for a couple of days, but your life is in danger if you go without breathing for just five minutes.

We don't normally pay special attention to breathing, because our bodies just do it on their own unless we consciously try to control it. It's similar to how we don't worry much about our body temperature. But although we always seem to be breathing the same way, in fact that's not the case. Our breathing is constantly changing, reflecting vital activity.

When we're young, the center of our breathing generally is close to the lower abdomen. It rises as we get older. Most adults move their chests more than their bellies when they breathe. We can also describe this by saying that our breathing becomes more shallow. In people who are sick and close to death, breathing is very shallow, barely getting past the throat. The shoulders move automatically to make this shallow breathing a little deeper. When breathing no longer goes beyond the throat, a person literally breathes his last.

The reason breathing is important for the recovery of natural healing ability is that it directly impacts the autonomic nervous system. It causes changes in other vital signs, too.

Try this experiment. With your hand on your opposite wrist or over your carotid artery just below your chin, slowly inhale and exhale. Feel how your pulse responds as you breathe in and out. You'll be able to feel your pulse slowing when you exhale, then quickening when you inhale. The quickening of your pulse is the action of the sympathetic nervous system, while the slowing is the action of the parasympathetic nervous system. In this way, respiration directly causes changes in vital signs—pulse, blood pressure, and body temperature—and also affects brain waves.

Breathing, pulse, blood pressure, and body temperature are all vital functions controlled by the autonomic nervous system. What makes breathing different from other functions is that, although it's automatic, it's the easiest to moderate intentionally. It's difficult to raise or lower blood pressure, pulse, or body temperature intentionally, but we can control them indirectly through our breathing. When breathing becomes deep, slow, and natural, the other vital signs recover balance. We might say that breathing is the master key to all our vital functions.

The body's physiological functions aren't the only things we can control through breathing. We can also control our emotions and thoughts. Can you become very, very angry while breathing very, very slowly? It's not possible. Our bodies and brains aren't built that way. When your breathing is controlled so that it becomes deeper and calmer, your thoughts grow quiet and your emotions settle down.

If you make good use of breathing in this way, you'll find it a powerful tool for regulating your thoughts and emotions. When you've been under stress, remember to take three deep breaths before saying or doing anything. Follow this simple rule, and you'll prevent yourself from saying, doing, and choosing many things that could cause you deep regrets later on.

When you feel rushed or angry, can't get to sleep, or are agitated, stop what you're doing for a moment to breathe slowly and deeply. Take just 10 breaths and your mind will become calm, your anger will subside, and you will feel peace. Breathing has great power.

BREATHING STRENGTHENS NATURAL HEALING POWER

Good, healthy breathing that contributes to the recovery of natural healing power is deep and slow, yet natural.

With one hand on your chest and the other on your lower abdomen, try to breathe naturally. Feel how you're breathing. Which moves more, your chest or your belly? If the hand on your chest moves more and your shoulders rise and fall, that's evidence that your breathing isn't deep. Commonly, the weaker your body and the more anxious your mind, the more you move your chest rather than your abdomen when you breathe.

The most important muscle for breathing is the diaphragm. Shaped like a dome, the diaphragm divides the thorax, where your lungs are located, from the abdomen, where your digestive organs are. Breathing happens with the rise and fall of the diaphragm, which draws breath in and pushes it out. The diaphragm is controlled by the abdominal muscles. When you push your lower abdomen forward, your diaphragm moves downward, increasing the volume of your lungs and drawing in a great deal of air.

Causing the diaphragm to move a bit lower not only has a positive effect on the abdominal organs, but it also greatly increases the volume of air accepted by the lungs. When the diaphragm is lowered just a centimeter, according to the American Lung Association (ALA), the lungs take in 250 to 300 cc more air. People who breathe deeply can lower their diaphragms about 4 cm, the ALA says, and take in more than 1,000 cc additional air every time they take a breath.

In order to breathe deeply, lower the center point of your breathing to your abdomen. In Asia since ancient times, people have not only considered breathing centered on the lower abdomen to be the secret to a long and healthy life, but they have also used it as an important way to develop concentration and elevate consciousness.

Placing one hand on the chest and the other on the lower abdomen while observing the movement of the belly is recommended for beginners as a deep-breathing practice. Inhale as you slowly press out your lower abdomen, concentrating your awareness there. Exhale slowly as you naturally relax your lower abdomen. Try to feel the movement of the hand on your stomach. As you continue to inhale and exhale with your lower abdomen, rhythmically repeat the movement of pushing out and relaxing your belly. Do this at a comfortable rate, but be sure to use a uniform rhythm as you extend and relax your lower abdomen. Inhalations and exhalations will continue naturally as your body and mind are in a comfortable state. When you inhale sufficiently, you exhale automatically, and once you've exhaled enough, you automatically take another breath. Practice this regularly and you'll be able to feel your breathing grow deeper as it gradually sinks from your chest to your lower abdomen.

Now let's attempt another experiment. Try to count your breaths. How many breaths do you take in a minute? Is your breathing fast or slow? For an adult, the optimal respiratory rate in a state of rest is once every 12 seconds, or five times a minute. Your cardiopulmonary efficiency will be maximized if you breathe at this rate.

If you breathe 7 to 10 times per minute, you are in a slightly excited state. Breathing 10 to 20 times indicates that you're in a stressed state of an intermediate level. More than 20 breaths per minute means that you are under considerable stress. Of course, there are exceptions to this general rule, but it's a well-known fact that the more relaxed our bodies and minds are, the more slowly we breathe.

Taking deep, slow breaths stimulates the parasympathetic nervous system. That elicits a relaxation response from the body, reducing everyday stress and stabilizing the mind. Conversely, habitually breathing quickly lowers the concentration of carbon dioxide in the blood, which causes the blood vessels to contract. Health is impacted as the level of oxygen sent to the body and brain drops.

The best way to breathe slowly is to be aware of your breathing. Simply being conscious of your breathing usually causes respiration to slow and deepen. The simplest and most effective way to do this is to count breaths. If other thoughts arise you'll lose count, so this is also good training for focusing the mind. At first it's not easy to count to a high number, so practice using a count of about 10. Inhaling and exhaling is one breathing cycle, so count this as one repetition. Repeat to a count of 10. Doing just three or four sets will cause your breath to automatically grow deeper and more natural. At the same time, you'll feel your mind becoming calmer and more peaceful.

Breathing can be a powerful means of restoring the autonomic nervous system to an appropriate state of balance. Frequency of breathing affects sympathetic dominance, and depth of breathing affects parasympathetic dominance. Accordingly, the most effective way to restore autonomic balance is to breathe slowly and deeply. Slow breathing calms an overly excited sympathetic nervous system; deep breathing strengthens a weary parasympathetic nervous system.

Good breathing is natural, deep, and slow. Respiration becomes gentle and deep at the same time. Unless breathing is deep, you can't take in enough oxygen to breathe slowly. Pay careful attention as you control your breathing and you'll be able to maximize your oxygen intake, increase your metabolism, and effectively expel waste material from your body.

As your breathing gradually deepens and slows, you'll feel the natural rhythm of life always flowing within you. And when your body's rhythm resonates with the rhythm of the great life force of the cosmos, your natural healing power starts to operate vigorously. Fill your body with the great life force of the universe as you take breaths deep into your lower abdomen. Send out all the stagnant energy in your body and mind as you exhale slowly. Your body and mind will recover their original balance and harmony as you breathe this way—deeply and slowly, yet naturally.

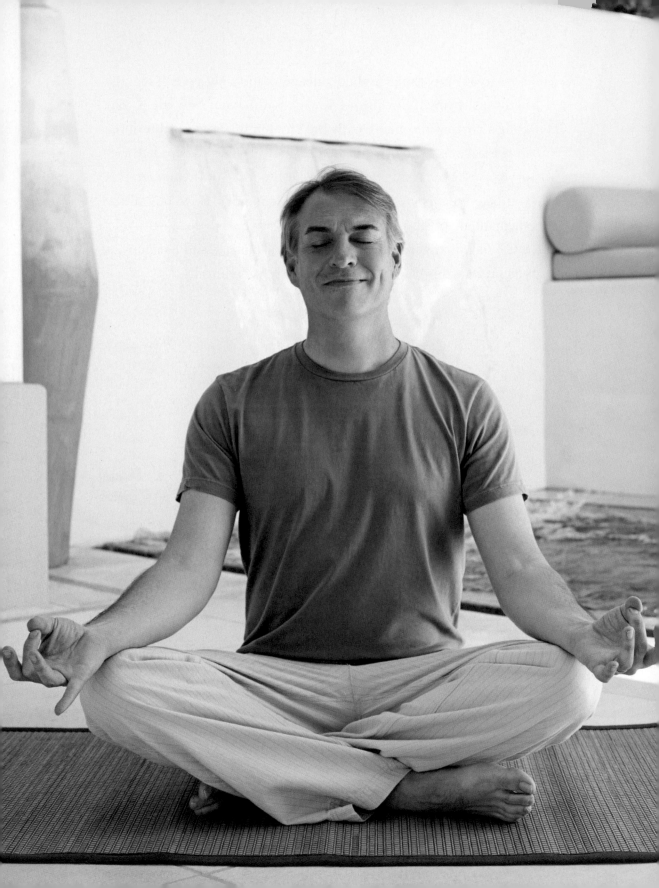

OBSERVE WITH YOUR MIND

THE MIND IS POWERFUL

Take three or four deep breaths and then try to relax your whole body comfortably. Now concentrate your awareness in the palm of one hand; it doesn't matter whether it's your left or your right hand. A concentration of awareness brings a concentration of energy, and a concentration of energy is manifest as a change in temperature. You can feel the temperature changing if you continue to focus, even for just a minute or two. Now bring the palms of your hands into contact with each other, and you can actually feel that the hand on which you focused has gotten warmer. Energy flows and blood concentrates where the mind directs it, causing heat to form. Our minds can actually create physical changes in our bodies.

You've probably heard about the placebo effect. This refers to what happens when illnesses are healed by autosuggestion, by a patient's belief that an ineffective substance is a real medication. Experiments have reportedly even shown that someone who has a serious allergic reaction to a certain kind of flower can have the same response to an artificial flower of that type. Our bodies respond to what we believe. This is such a widespread phenomenon that the placebo test is essential for newly developed drugs to earn recognition. And countless drugs fail this test—they can't get recognition as being significantly more effective than a fake drug. Product development is discontinued as a result.

Mainstream medicine still views the placebo effect as an incidental, fascinating fact caused by an illusion of the mind. But if we examine this from a different perspective, we see that the medicine of belief is the most powerful medicine of all. The mind has greater power than we might imagine. In particular, it exerts a great influence on health, positive or negative.

What thought is passing through your mind right now? What emotion? Countless emotions arise as a consequence of a single thought, and these cause a variety of chemical, physiological changes in our bodies. When you think joyful thoughts, happy hormones such as serotonin and dopamine are secreted in your body; if you hold negative feelings too long, stress hormones such as cortisol and epinephrine are secreted.

Let's say you've come home feeling refreshed after doing weight training for an hour at the gym, working up a great sweat. Or you've come home in the best state of positive energy, feeling like everything in the world exists for you, after spending an hour at a yoga studio. And let's say that, unfortunately, that evening you have a huge fight with your spouse or child, without making up. Could you maintain a positive energy state and peace of mind even then? Most people would probably not get much sleep, their minds awash in all kinds of thoughts and emotions. Your breathing probably will become irregular, your head get hot, your neck and shoulders stiffen from stress, and your lower abdomen, hands, and feet grow cold.

Trying to govern your health only by exercise and by what you eat and drink, without controlling your thoughts and emotions, is like trying to keep your computer in good shape by managing the hardware but not the software. So it's important to realize that your thoughts and emotions are things you can choose, not something outside your control. While thoughts may arise without your choosing them, like breezes blowing in from somewhere unknown, the way you respond to them is entirely up to you.

It's not easy to control your mind as you desire, but it's definitely not impossible. You simply need practice. Just as we practice controlling body temperature and breathing to recover natural healing power, so, too, we can practice controlling our thoughts and emotions—the contents of our minds. There is nothing in the world that doesn't get better with practice.

MY EMOTIONS ARE MINE, BUT NOT ME

How can you use the power of your mind to control your thoughts and emotions? The most powerful means is by observation—in other words, by watching. Observation is the most essential and powerful ability that the mind has. There is nothing in this world, from tangible things like trees and stones to intangibles like thoughts and emotions, that doesn't become an object of observation when we calm and focus our minds. If there's something you're having trouble observing, it's because your mind isn't clear and calm enough to manifest that ability, not because of a limit on the mind's ability.

The mind that lucidly watches its thoughts and emotions without chasing after them, or intentionally ignoring or denying them, causes them to evaporate like fog in sunlight. All the training methods we usually call "meditation" have this kind of observation at their core, regardless of any technical or methodological differences.

The most powerful change in perception we can experience through observation is that we can see ourselves as separate from our experiences. This means that we observe our sensations, thoughts, and emotions as objects, instead of identifying ourselves with them. Suppose your boss makes you angry, and you have the thought, *My boss is a real jerk*. Rather than identifying with that thought, you could simply tell yourself that you have that thought. When you're angry because of the thought, rather than saying to yourself, *I'm angry*, you could say, *I have anger right now*.

In that moment, thought and feeling become objects separated from your mind. You become able to make a wiser, more considerate choice instead of acting in a way that's dictated by a negative thought or feeling.

This also goes for the pains and diseases of the body. If I'm suffering from a tumor in my lungs, instead of identifying myself with a body that has a tumor, I can objectify my body. When I identify myself with my body, I may experience negative emotions about the pain and prognosis from the tumor, such as fear, anger, and frustration. Once I'm able to objectify my body, however, such emotions change into compassion, and the mind has sympathy for the one suffering. An energy of unconditional love toward the suffering object—the energy of fundamental healing flowing beneath all vital phenomena—starts to flow from this compassion.

I'm in the habit of advising people to repeat out loud the following two affirmations as a way to develop their mental power to observe phenomena arising in their bodies and minds without identifying themselves with them. "My body is not me, but mine. My emotions are not me, but mine." When your body causes you to suffer, when you're confused and swept away by an intense whirlwind of thoughts and emotions, try to focus your attention and repeat these two affirmations. Try saying them out loud right now. "My body is not me, but mine. My emotions are not me, but mine."

You will discover the strength to return to a calm, solid center even amid all the human emotions of your life, the power to recover harmony even amid all the changes and uncertainties of life, the power to restore ceaseless passion and hope for life even amid all kinds of trial and error, failure, and frustration. That power is your natural healing ability—the great life force of the cosmos, the solar energy I continually emphasize in this book.

The mind that quietly watches all the thoughts and emotions arising within it without becoming attached to any of them has the power to return everything to a state of balance—its natural state. That is why I consider the observing mind to be the third key to restoring natural healing ability.

WHEN YOUR MIND OBSERVES YOUR TEMPERATURE AND BREATHING

As quantum physics explains to us, the observation of the conscious mind has the power to create and maintain physical phenomena. What is created depends on the state and intentions of the observing mind. A mind that is detached and clear, without greed or fear, has the power to restore its object of observation to its original, natural state. This applies to vital phenomena such as body temperature or breathing, too. Body heat, mindful breathing, and observation with the mind—in combination, these have an amazing power to restore an unbalanced autonomic nervous system to a healthy state of parasympathetic dominance.

When you feel your body in a state of mental calm and physical comfort, you'll begin to feel your body heat. The first reason we have trouble feeling our body heat in our everyday lives is that our consciousness is turned toward the outside. We don't have the time to feel what's inside us when our head is a tangle of thoughts and emotions. It's not easy to feel body heat even when our heads aren't in such a jumble. That's because our temperature-sensing nerves, being a part of our bodies, have a temperature similar to the rest of our bodies. It's like what happens if you immerse your body in water that's close to your body temperature. The sensation of having a body disappears, and you seem to melt into the water.

Being able to feel your body temperature requires a depth of concentration. Subtle changes in body temperature and in the temperature balance between head and lower abdomen result from the concentration of the focused mind. Consequently, the calm and focused mind detects those changes. This itself is already a deep state of meditation. There is no one who doesn't meditate while sensing the temperature in his or her own body, especially in an ordinary state when the body is neither hot nor cold. Whether it's intentional or not, feeling your body temperature means that you are already in a state of deep meditation.

A surprising and important change happens at this time: the object of observation begins to change. Observation starts with your breath and body heat, but while you're relaxed and concentrating on your breathing and body temperature, your observing mind itself becomes the object of observation. And as your very mind becomes the object of observation, its remaining thoughts and emotions vanish, regardless of your intentions. The vicious cycle of stress-causing thoughts and emotions is broken while the mind observes itself.

In this way, breathing and body temperature can be the switch that turns on the observing mind, while at the same time they are the objects that this mind observes and changes. When you observe your breathing, it automatically deepens and slows, and when you observe your body temperature, it recovers a healthy rhythm, range, and balance. Through this process, you create an optimal state in which your natural healing ability can manifest its power. And as your mind itself becomes the object of your observation, your thoughts and emotions are calmed, your stress-reaction mode is shut down, and your healing mode is turned on.

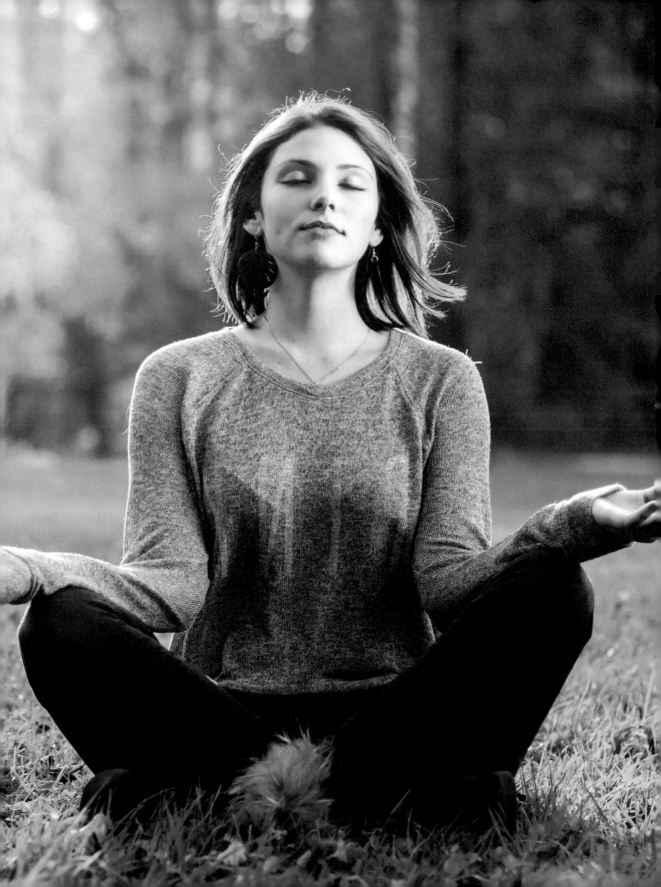

CHAPTER 2

THE **SOLAR BODY** METHOD

WHAT IS A SOLAR BODY?

EMBRACING THE SUN IN YOUR BODY

In the previous chapter, I introduced the concept of natural healing power and spoke about body temperature, breathing, and the observing mind as the three keys for restoring our bodies' natural healing power. But recovering natural healing power doesn't mean simply developing resistance to disease. The natural healing power of which I speak has a much deeper and more fundamental meaning.

Recovering natural healing power means regaining a connection with the infinite life force of the cosmos. It is discovering the essence of who you really are, not hurt by anything and remaining changeless even amid innumerable changes. The natural healing power about which I speak, in that sense, includes a spiritual dimension.

The greatest change that you experience when you've recovered natural healing power is that you come to have a self-reliant, self-sustaining perspective toward life. You're transformed from depending on the outside for your health and happiness to creating these things for yourself. You live truly as the master of your life, trusting in the great restorative power of the life inside you.

I had been trying to think of an appropriate term to express this powerful and beautiful transformation. One day during meditation, I found one that captured my mind—"Solar Body." A Solar Body is someone who recovers natural healing power and the goodness of human nature to create her own health and happiness. Solar Body came to me as a kind of inspiration, but I have various reasons for using the sun as a comparison for people who have bright, healthy bodies and minds.

The sun is the fundamental and essential energy source through which all life-forms on the earth can live. The light of the sun heats the ground and the sea. It creates the wind by causing differences in temperature in the atmosphere. Not only does it perform the physical work of circulating water, but it also serves as life energy, causing all life-forms to exist and grow. We may forget to feel gratitude for the sun because solar energy, like air, can be had so easily for free. But just as humans cannot live more than a few minutes without air, so we cannot imagine humans—or the earth—existing without the sun.

The solar energy I'm experiencing with my body right now isn't all that comes from the sun. Plants make carbohydrates by using sunlight for photosynthesis, and animals and humans use those carbohydrates as an energy source. Every living thing contains solar energy. Solar energy makes the whole world go round and round. Even the petroleum and coal we use for heating our houses and moving our machines is solar energy accumulated over hundreds of millions of years.

The heart of natural healing ability is a state of physical and mental vitality created by developing an energy center in the lower abdomen, and by maintaining an energy balance—the head cool and the lower abdomen warm. This is like holding the sun in your belly. A person with a Solar Body overflows with health and vitality, and with bright, warm life energy.

Like the sun—the only body in our solar system that gives off its own light and heat—a Solar Body is someone who can manage the infinite energy source within him. The important point is that Solar Bodies can do this for themselves. Not depending on experts or external sources, they know how to make their own bodies and minds overflow with vitality, and they constantly put this knowledge into practice.

A MIND SHINING LIKE THE SUN

A Solar Body doesn't only have physical health and vitality. It expresses mental health—in other words, recovery of the goodness of human nature. According to a passage in an ancient Korean scripture, the ChunBuKyung, "Our original mind is bright like the sun, and seeks its own brightness." Our original mind is the intrinsic essence of mind, the true self. In Eastern traditions, it comes before thought, desire, any conceptualization at all. That is our finest essence, which is inherently pure and good.

The mind within us that is bright like the sun is our true nature and the substance of our humanity. It is the natural power that heals our physical diseases and returns us to a balanced state, the compassion that causes us to feel sympathy when we see suffering people, and the absolute mirror within us. It is our conscience, which lets us know that we are true when we are true and that we are false when we are false. Although it appears at times as natural healing power, at other times as compassion, and sometimes as conscience and wisdom, its source is one. It is the sun within us, our true nature. Realizing this is very important, for once you've encountered this mind within you, you want it. You develop the will to seek it if you've lost it.

The mind within us, shining brilliantly like the sun, can be described as the "soul" or "divinity." Our emotions and environments change ceaselessly, just as the seasons and weather change, but that mind is always shining there, like the sun. When you feel that mind shining within you, you develop an attitude of appreciation for your own nobility. And when you consider yourself precious and noble, you develop the same attitude toward other life, and to the world.

To have a Solar Body is to switch from a life dependent on externalities for health and happiness to a life lived creating your own health and happiness. The causes and the answers are to be found within yourself. Whatever situation you face, don't look for the cause elsewhere, but think, *I've caused the present situation.* This is not victim consciousness, but is about taking greater ownership of your life. If you feel that someone else created your problems, you have to wait for others to come and solve them. But when you search for the causes within yourself, you'll see the solutions. You'll have the will to solve your problems yourself, and you'll actively look for ways to do so.

Having a Solar Body also means recovering the connection with your soul that you may have lost. It's about living a meaningful life and bringing that life into full bloom no matter what your circumstances may be, with absolute faith and trust in the power of that great life within you.

In our busy, driven lives, we have almost no time to reflect on the nature of our original mind. And even if we do have the time, finding and maintaining that reflective attitude isn't easy. But no matter how depressed or wearied we may be by the ups and downs of life, the ChunBuKyung teaches us that if we go to the very bottom of our minds, there we will find the original mind, shining brilliantly like the sun.

We all have an original mind that is bright like the sun. Those who discover theirs and shine its light on all around them, those whose bodies and minds overflow with life energy just as the powerful sun emits solar energy—these are Solar Bodies.

In my book *Change: Realizing Your Great Potential*, I stressed that genuine change is possible only when we become one with the whole that transcends our individuality, with the power that binds and connects all things, with our true essence, changeless even amid change. About 30 years ago, I experienced this wholeness with my entire body. I felt myself transcending the boundaries of my physical body to expand to infinity, and this has been described as a very bright light and hot heat. This isn't my experience alone. In all times and places, most significant spiritual experiences have been accompanied by feelings of light, heat, and infinite expansion.

The expression I use in this book, *solar energy*, in a certain context does mean energy coming directly from the sun. But in a more fundamental sense, it indicates this wholeness that transcends our individuality, this power flowing as one in all things in existence.

Solar energy is experienced in our bodies as feelings of energetic warmth and expansiveness. But becoming a Solar Body isn't about passively experiencing this warm and expansive energy. It's about generating it yourself and sharing it actively with others.

THE SOLAR BODY METHOD

Now it's time to introduce in earnest a method for creating a Solar Body. The Solar Body Method is made up of three principal components—Sunlight Meditation, Solar Energy Circuit Training, and Solar Body Exercises. Each of these in itself is a wonderful exercise for restoring natural healing power, but the effects are multiplied when the practices are combined.

- **Sunlight Meditation** involves receiving solar energy directly through sunlight. It's a way of exposing your body to sunlight and receiving the solar energy contained in sunlight and circulating it throughout your body.

  Anyone can easily practice this method in a place well lit by the sun. Whenever you get a chance to go outdoors, try to accept warm solar energy with your whole body through Sunlight

Meditation. You can even use this form of meditation while going for a walk.

- **Solar Energy Circuit Training** is the heart of the Solar Body Method. It involves charging yourself with solar energy by using 12 energy circuits based on the patterns in which cosmic energy moves. This can maximize natural healing power by using your consciousness to powerfully change and amplify your body's energy phenomena in a very short period of time.

  The process might feel a little strange and difficult at first if you haven't had previous experience with energy training, but in fact it's an easy practice requiring no special techniques. The effects are unimaginably rapid and powerful if you open your heart so that the solar energy coming in through the circuits can act on your body and mind.

- **Solar Body Exercises** provide a means of increasing body temperature through simple movements and restoring optimal energy balance—the head cool and the belly warm. The three exercises are so simple that they take only a few minutes to learn, but their effects are so outstanding that countless people worldwide have effectively and amazingly recovered their health through them.

- As a support for the Solar Body Method, I'm also introducing the use of what I call the **solar herb—sage**. Sage has strong healing ingredients, and chewing on fresh sage leaves as described later in this book will maximize its healing effects.

The ideal way to use the Solar Body Method is to open the energy channels in your body through the three Solar Body Exercises and then do Solar Energy Circuit Training. It's even better if you can do your Solar Energy Circuit Training outdoors, letting you accept sunlight with your whole body.

By practicing the Solar Body Method, you'll find that the three keys for recovering natural healing power—body temperature, breathing, and observation of the mind—will happen automatically and together, even without having that as your goal. You will come to understand what this means as you follow the Solar Body Method.

SUNLIGHT MEDITATION

THE GIFT GIVEN BY THE SUN

All organisms on earth live on energy from the sun, and human beings are no exception. We're influenced indirectly through the food we eat—plants and animals that have grown on solar energy—but our bodies are also directly influenced by the sunlight pouring down on us. Infrared light warms us and visible light lets us see objects. Ultraviolet light disinfects us and generates vitamin D in our bodies.

Vitamin D has such a positive effect on our natural healing power that we can consider it a gift from the sun. Vitamin D not only makes our bones strong and prevents osteoporosis by increasing the absorption rate of calcium, but it is thought to be effective for diabetes, periodontitis, multiple sclerosis, and cancer—especially prostate cancer, breast cancer, and intestinal cancer. The incidence of prostate cancer is said to be approximately 50 percent higher in males who are deficient in vitamin D.

The key is getting enough sunshine, since we don't get enough vitamin D in our diets. About 15 minutes of sunlight a day fills our daily requirement. People in rural environments reportedly get twice as much vitamin D as city-dwellers.

Sunlight also promotes secretion of melatonin, the hormone that contributes to a good night's sleep. Serotonin, the "happiness hormone," is also secreted in greater quantities after exposure to sunlight. Serotonin promotes feelings of well-being as the mind becomes stable, while not having enough of it leads to anxiety, nervousness, and depression. Low levels of melatonin and serotonin because of decreased sunlight is considered a major cause of wintertime seasonal affective disorder (SAD). The best way to overcome this is by getting a certain amount of sunlight every day. Higher levels of serotonin also help control appetite, while lower levels stimulate appetite and contribute to overeating.

Sunlight is essential for increasing body temperature, too. Our body temperature drops to its lowest during the night and rises during the day, when we're active. The more active we are in sunlight, especially outdoors, the higher our body temperature rises. If your hands and feet feel cold and your body temperature has dropped, try sitting for just 10 minutes in bright sunlight. You'll quickly feel your body heating up and even your hands and feet growing warmer.

Being exposed to very strong sunlight for too long can be damaging to your body because of the intense ultraviolet light. You want to do your training in the right intensity of sunlight, but that varies according to the season, weather, and time of day. In the middle of the summer, when the weather is humid, avoid the times when sunlight is hottest. Conversely, in cold winter choose the time when sunlight is most intense, around noon. And while sunrise and sunset are good times for Sunlight Meditation, the intensity of the light is a little weak then for increasing body temperature. Depending on the season and the climate, between 9 and 11 a.m. and between 2 and 5 p.m. generally are good times.

Ultraviolet B, which synthesizes vitamin D, is almost completely filtered from sunlight that comes in through a glass window. If you want to recharge in a sunlit room, open a window so the light hits you directly. It's also good to wear clothing made of thin material so sunlight reaches your skin, and to expose some parts of your body—your face, arms, and legs—directly to the sunlight.

In the summer when sunlight is intense, just five minutes could be enough. When sunlight is weak and body temperature drops in the winter, be sure to get at least 20 minutes of exposure so your body can heat up sufficiently. Your body will signal when it's sufficiently charged—you'll feel a tingling to the ends of your fingers and toes. Rising body temperature makes your blood vessels expand, promoting energy and blood flow. It's good to end your training when you get that feeling. Continuing too long could have an adverse effect: your body could overheat, and ultraviolet light could cause excessive production of harmful free oxygen radicals.

Promote energy and blood circulation by charging yourself with solar energy at least once a day, or once in the morning and again in the afternoon. Once you're surrounded by warm, bright sunlight and the cold, moist energy has left your body, your mind becomes peaceful as the worries in your head disappear. Your body and mind relax, stabilizing your brain waves so that drowsiness comes over you. Charged with solar energy, your lower abdomen, hands, and feet grow warm—a feeling that lasts for several hours.

When your hands or feet are cold or the energy of your body and mind feels dark, go out into the sunlight. Solar energy will gradually drive away the dark, cold energy and you will feel refreshed soon.

HOW TO DO
THE SUNLIGHT MEDITATION

No special technique is needed to receive the gift of sunlight. All you have to do is adopt whatever posture is comfortable for you—lying, sitting, or standing—and enjoy your fill of warm sunlight. However, you can recharge even more effectively if you induce the flow of energy through specific postures and focused awareness.

HOW TO GET SOLAR ENERGY
FACING THE SUN

1. Facing the sun, sit in a chair or on the floor in a half-lotus posture with your lower back straight. Place your hands on your knees, palms facing up, and relax your chest and shoulders. Close your eyes and smile very slightly.

2. Enjoy the sunlight pouring down on your whole body. Imagining your body to be a solar panel, visualize receiving and being charged with energy. Move your awareness down your body—from face to shoulders, arms, chest, abdomen, and legs—imagining warm sunshine melting each part in turn.

3. Lifting your head slightly, commune with the solar energy shining down on your face. As you very slowly turn your head

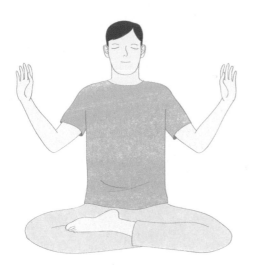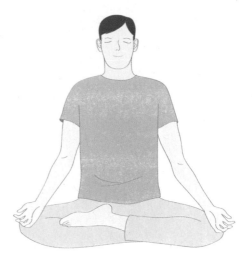

from side to side, try to feel the colors of light changing before your closed eyes. When you face the sun you'll sense a bright golden light, and when you turn slightly to the side you'll perceive oranges and reds. Commune with the solar energy in the colors.

4. Stop moving your head and receive the solar energy coming into your face, into your whole body. Store it in your lower abdomen—in your "energy center." Keep visualizing as you feel your lower abdomen growing warmer. End the training when you feel that your whole body, including fingers and toes, has been warmed sufficiently.

HOW TO GET SOLAR ENERGY
FACING AWAY FROM THE SUN

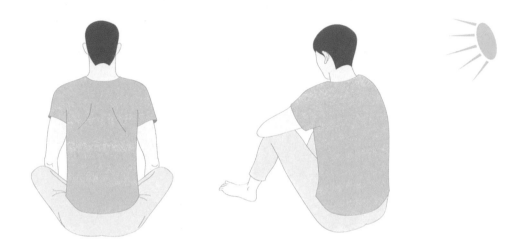

1. With your back to the sun, sit sideways in a chair or in a half-lotus posture on the floor, or in some other comfortable posture. It's OK to bend your head and your body forward slightly so that sunlight touches your entire back.

2. Imagine that your back is a solar panel and accept the solar energy entering it. Feel your shoulders, lungs, kidneys, and lower back gradually grow warmer. Imagine solar energy filling your lungs, driving out the cold and wet energy that causes all sorts of respiratory diseases.

3. Feel the heat being amplified in your lower abdomen as you visualize filling it with the solar energy entering through your back. End the training when you feel that your whole body, including fingers and toes, has been warmed sufficiently.

PRECAUTIONS OF SUNLIGHT MEDITATION

Exposing yourself to sunlight for too long is absolutely to be avoided. It's important to prevent your body from overheating by ending the training once you feel that your whole body, including your hands and feet, is warm enough. Especially avoid overexposing yourself to intense summer sunlight. Your core temperature could rise too far, resulting in rapid heartbeat, headache, and dizziness.

Replenish your body moisture by drinking plenty of water before and after this training. Lukewarm rather than cold water is best. For outdoor activities that involve major exertion, like hiking or mountain climbing, drink water before you start out and then drink more at 15-minute intervals to replenish the moisture your body loses through sweat while you're active.

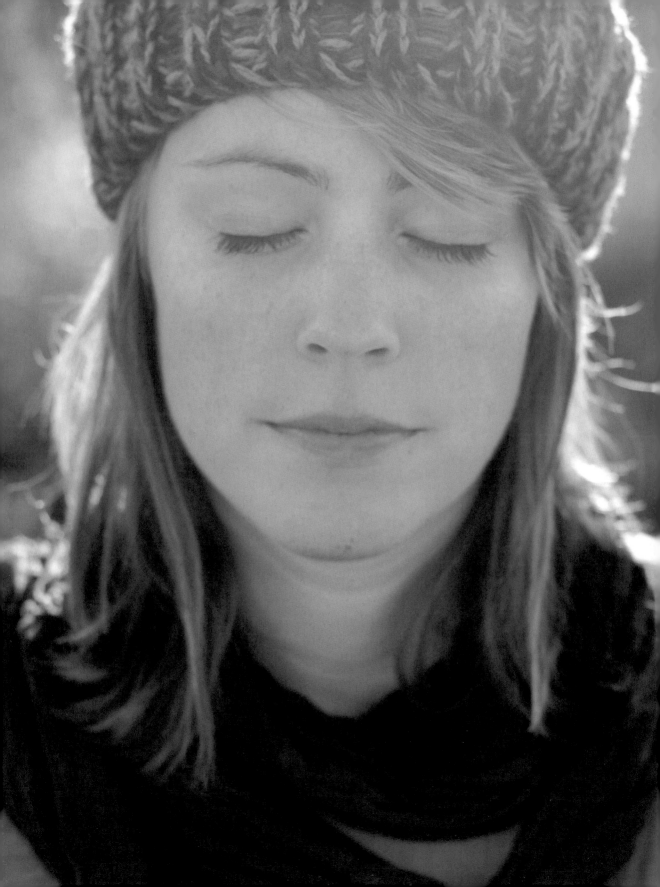

SOLAR ENERGY CIRCUIT TRAINING

TWO PRINCIPLES FOR GENERATING ENERGY

I've talked about receiving solar energy directly from sunlight. But even without sunlight, it's possible to generate body heat and energy for the recovery of natural healing power. Solar Energy Circuit Training is just for that.

It's important to understand two basic principles for generating energy with this specific training. The first principle is that *specific forms create specific energies*. In other words, whether it's a point, a line, or a three-dimensional form, everything with shape and color has a corresponding energy.

Place a blank sheet of paper in front of you right now. What feeling do you get when you look at it? Now draw a triangle on the paper. How are the feelings you have when you look at the triangle different from when you looked at the blank sheet of paper? Feelings are energy. The energy you feel in the triangle will be different from the energy you feel in blank paper. Now draw a square and a circle. How are the feelings you get from those shapes different from what you get from the triangle?

Everything that has a shape gives us a different feeling, and those feelings are perceived by our brains as specific energies. Consequently, circuits composed of lines of different shapes generate specific energies.

We can consciously create or amplify those energies through the power of imagination—that is, the power of the mind. The second principle is that *the mind creates energy.*

As modern quantum physics is revealing, nothing in the universe is fixed and unchanging. From our rotating spiral galaxy to the microscopic cells in the human body, everything is made up of restlessly vibrating elementary particles. If we were to look at this whole world through a high-performance microscope that allowed us to perceive elementary particles, we'd see that nothing stands still and everything is vibrating.

One of the important discoveries of quantum physics is that elementary particles can take the form of either waves or particles, depending on the mind of the observer. In other words, our minds—becoming energy—can impact reality, the material world.

By combining the two principles—"Specific forms create specific energies" and "The mind creates energy"—I have devised Solar Energy Circuit Training. In other words, this is a method for activating, through the concentration of awareness, circuits that can positively change and amplify the flow of energy in our bodies.

We are not beings separated from the energy of the cosmos. Humans ceaselessly exchange their energy with that of the cosmos, as do all beings in the world. Our bodies could be called energy bodies that vibrate ceaselessly beyond the physical dimension visible to the eyes. Countless elementary particles are vibrating subtly in the tens of trillions of cells in the human body. Although this occurs throughout the body, the channels in which energy circulation is particularly vigorous are called "energy meridians," and the places where energy pools (or enters or exits the body) are called "meridian points." Our bodies are known to have 12 major meridians and more than 360 meridian points. The flow and balance of energy is regulated through the system of chakras, or energy centers.

This occurs spontaneously, even if we're not necessarily aware of the details. What's truly important, however, is that we can consciously change and amplify the energy phenomena of the human body. And we can experience this instantaneously through the concentration of our awareness—in other words, through imagination and visualization, rather than through physical movements such as yoga or stretching.

Just as current flows if you move a coiled magnet, we can generate currents and energy as we wish by causing an energy circuit to pass through or rotate in our bodies. As cosmic life force flows through the energy circuits, they generate heat, and the energy moves more vigorously, greatly amplifying its waves.

MY SOLAR ENERGY CIRCUIT STORY

One day when I was meditating outdoors, I opened my eyes and saw the energy of the sun intermingling with particles of air. I noticed that the sun's energy traveled in waves of varying lengths and vibrations—differing stitches in the tapestry of energy that, at surface level, we call sunlight. I watched as many different patterns, or wave forms, traveled through the air and were absorbed by plant life, by my body, and even by the rocks around me. Everything received the energy patterns of the sun and was enlivened by them.

I began to play with those different patterns, seeing what effect each one had on my nervous system, my energy system, even my body. I realized that the complete energy of the sun may sustain life on this planet, but the individual waves could be used as tools for producing various effects in a damaged or incomplete energy system.

Inspired by the changes that I perceived in my own body, with the power of my mind I began to intentionally generate certain wave forms and to use them as instruments to facilitate healing in others. I discovered a pattern. Certain wave forms could be used to produce certain results, and a combination of forms could become a recipe for recovering our natural healing power.

Based on the energy patterns I saw in the sunlight—and on my own experiences, research, and application on other people over the years—I have systematized the patterns of cosmic life energy entering our bodies into 12 different solar energy circuits. Now I am sharing what I have learned with you, like a prescription for using the sun's energy as a natural medicine.

HOW DO SOLAR ENERGY CIRCUITS WORK?

People commonly experience increased heat and more vigorous energy waves in their bodies when they do Solar Energy Circuit Training. It's similar to what you feel when you get solar energy directly through sunlight. Later, when you're familiar with this training, you'll feel yourself being charged much more powerfully and rapidly than from sunlight alone.

What's important is concentrating your awareness, maximizing your use of the power of your mind. If you think, *I don't seem to be doing this training well,* you'll only be able to experience that much energy. If you think, *I can get incredible energy through this training,* you'll be able to draw powerful energy into yourself. I'll say it again: consciousness and energy are not separate. Consciousness creates energy, and energy creates consciousness. The two always react to and influence each other.

The greater the strength of your mind, the more rapidly solar energy rotates, charging your body. The speed of light is known to be the speed limit of the universe. Nothing, they say, can move faster than light. Light is fast, but it still takes time for it to move, because it's a physical entity. It takes about eight minutes for light from the sun to reach the earth, but it takes an incredible 2.3 million years for that light to travel to Andromeda, the galaxy closest to our own. Viewed on a cosmic scale, light isn't all that fast! However, the speed of our minds has no limits at all. The speed of your mind is merely restricted by the limits you've set for yourself. Repeat this Solar Energy Circuit Training for a while, and you'll experience just how powerful your mind can be.

When your training deepens, you'll be able to generate in a minute heat like you'd experience after 10 to 20 minutes under the sun. Although the sensation may be small at first, if you concentrate on that feeling as you continue training, your focus will improve, and eventually you'll be able to experience intense heat and light. Then you can instantly charge yourself with solar energy by concentrating your awareness anywhere and anytime, even during sunless nights or cloudy days, or indoors.

With that level of focus, you will be able to feel specific circuits being applied in a concentrated way to your body, especially in your neck, chest, legs, and specific organs. As the circuits rapidly pass through certain parts of your body, you'll feel cold energy leaving, a stinging feeling entering, and a very hot feeling spreading. Small or large vibrations may actually occur in your body, depending on the intensity of a circuit's application. As the circuits' current passes through you, it causes a contraction of muscles. The current intensifies as blockages to energy flow are removed. It's as if someone was stepping on a water hose turned on at full blast and then suddenly released it, causing the hose to shake wildly. As with the hose, the vibrations will calm when your energy flows more smoothly and softly.

Emotional effects also result as your energy becomes bright like the sun. Feelings of sadness or anger will naturally be replaced with joy and happiness. Your body and mind will develop a sensation of lightness. In the process, you may even find yourself weeping, coughing, yawning, burping, etc. Don't try to control the physical and emotional phenomena you experience. Instead, just entrust your body to the sensation. With your relaxed focus and acceptance, natural healing will occur and the stagnant and cold energy will automatically leave your body.

Through Solar Energy Circuit Training, you'll be able to experience the three conditions of natural healing—body temperature, breathing, and observation of the mind—occurring automatically. As the application of the circuits gradually grows more intense, your body temperature will rise, but you'll recover a natural balance of temperature and energy, with your head growing cooler and your abdomen warmer. Your breathing may be rapid at first as you experience subtle or intense vibrations, but later it will become even, slow, and stable.

You will gain a deeper understanding of the relationship between mind and energy as you observe diverse energy phenomena arising in your body and your mind. In the instant we open our minds and accept solar energy with our whole bodies, we automatically create an environment capable of maximizing natural healing power.

BASIC TRAINING FOR SOLAR ENERGY CIRCUITS

Before you begin working with the 12 circuits, it's a good idea to start with some basic training in order to experience how specific circuits amplify energy, and how the mind can generate energy.

When you are connected with a circuit, you can feel various energy sensations such as warmth, coldness, tingling, pulsation, or vibration. You can continue the training as long as you want, but I suggest 5 to 10 minutes for each session.

In the beginning, do one circuit per training session. Later, once you get familiar with the training, you can combine as many circuits into one session as you want.

BASIC TRAINING 1: CIRCUIT COMING DOWN THROUGH THE HANDS

Sitting on the floor in a half-lotus posture or in a chair, straighten your spine. Relax your shoulders and hold your hands, palms up, about 5 or 6 inches above your knees. Gently close your eyes and focus your mind on the palms of your hands. Now concentrate on the very center of your palms.

Visualize pillars of golden solar energy coming down into the middle of your palms and into your hands. Your hands will

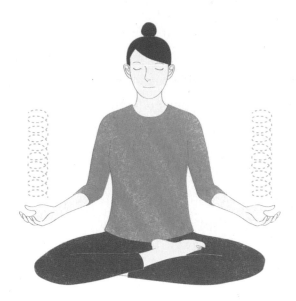

gradually feel heavier. Slowly lift your hands up about 2 inches and then lower them again, repeating this motion as you feel a sense of weight in your hands. That heaviness or tingling sensation is the feeling of energy.

Slowly stop your movements, and now visualize a spiral of solar energy whirling rapidly into the center of your palms. Focus your awareness, imagining the spiral circuit entering your palms powerfully and rapidly. Imagine this circuit breaking through blockages in your energy pathways as it travels along your arms to your elbows and shoulders. Your hands will gradually grow warmer, and they may experience large or subtle vibrations.

Traveling along your arms and into your body, the two circuits will meet in your chest, filling it with bright light.

Observe the energy state of your body after the training. You'll breathe more comfortably with your chest, heat will be generated in your arms and chest, and you'll be able to feel the waves and movements of energy in your body amplified. Inhale deeply and then exhale slowly as you end your training.

BASIC TRAINING 2: CIRCUIT COMING DOWN THROUGH THE SPINE

Sitting on the floor in a half-lotus posture or in a chair, straighten your spine. With shoulders and chest relaxed, place your hands on your knees, palms up. Tuck in your chin slightly so that your spine and head form a straight line. Gently close your eyes and concentrate on the crown of your head, where a powerful energy point is located. You'll feel the energy point better if you tap the crown of your head with the index and middle finger of one hand repeatedly 10 to 20 times.

Now imagine a spiral of golden solar energy circulating clockwise, descending into the crown of your head from somewhere above. This spiral circuit enters your head and, passing your brain, descends into your spine. The circuit rotates rapidly and powerfully in a spiral shape, creating an energy channel as it passes each joint of your spine.

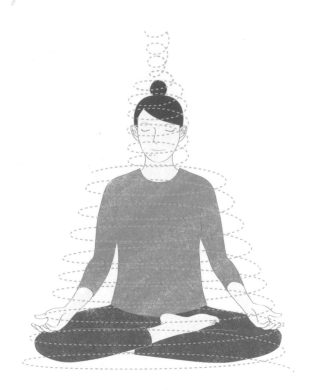

The radius of the spiral now expands so that the energy coils around your trunk. Your head may move back and forth, or you may experience large or small vibrations centered on your spine. Your body is enveloped in a space where this spiral form vibrates at high speed. The solar energy filling that space charges your body.

Observe your energy state after the circuit training. Heat will be generated in your body, especially in your lower abdomen, and your chest will feel lighter, your mind brighter, and your body's energy waves amplified. Inhale deeply, exhale slowly, and end the training.

BASIC TRAINING 3: CIRCUIT APPROACHING THE THIRD EYE

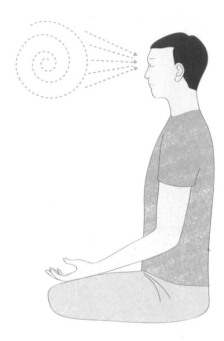

Sitting on the floor in a half-lotus posture or in a chair, straighten your spine. With your shoulders and chest relaxed, place your hands on your knees, palms up. Tuck in your chin slightly so that your spine and head form a straight line. Gently close your eyes.

Focus your mind on your third eye, the energy point in the center of your forehead. Imagine light spiraling clockwise before your eyes as it approaches you. Those who have sufficiently activated energy in their third eye will be able to see that light. But if you don't see it, it's enough just to imagine the light.

Imagine the spiral of energy entering your third eye and spreading throughout your brain and body. You may feel as if the light is approaching you or as if you're gradually entering more deeply into that light. Visualize your whole body shining brightly through the light.

Observe your energy state after the circuit training. Heat will be generated in your body, your head will feel refreshed, and you'll feel that your body's energy waves have been amplified. Inhale deeply, exhale slowly, and end the training.

SOLAR ENERGY CIRCUIT TRAINING, **STEP BY STEP**

The following 12 energy circuits, representing the complete energy of the sun, can be classified in four categories for natural healing: Circulation, Power, Creation, and Completion. I suggest that you begin at Level 1, the circulation circuits, and familiarize yourself with each one. Practice all of them before you move on to the next level. Completing the levels in order will let you fully integrate the vibration of each circuit into your energy field, giving you time to master each circuit successively. After you are accustomed to each circuit, you can freely combine different circuits in different orders or use the 12 circuits all at once.

Once you're familiar with the feelings and operations of these circuits in your body, you can use them for various tasks you have to accomplish in your life, or for goals you want to achieve. You can call on them to deliver energy to others who need help or healing by mentally focusing on those you want to help. You can apply them to eliminate or change problems or negative thoughts, emotions, or memories. You can deliver positive energy through the circuits to focus on personal goals, and to increase the power of your actions to achieve those goals.

The possibilities are open to you. The more familiar you become with the 12 solar energy circuits, the greater and brighter will grow the energy available for your use—and the greater will be the creativity you are able to manifest

FOR **EACH** CIRCUIT

Circuit training at any level involves a process of attunement, connecting, and channeling energy. The basic approach is the same for any circuit. These three steps will help you become comfortable with each new solar energy circuit that you use:

1. Sketch the circuit on a piece of paper.
2. Draw the circuit in the air with your hand.
3. Connect the circuit through your whole body by means of intention, visualization, and observation of the sensations in your body while you're working with the circuit.

- **To begin, sit in a comfortable position** with your back as straight as possible. If this posture is difficult for you, you can lie flat on your back. You can also take a standing position, if you'd like. A straight spine is important because it stacks the chakra line, ensuring that energy can flow without interruption. You can rock your hips from side to side to relieve any pressure in your spine.

- **To bring yourself into the present** so that you can access the infinite energy available to you, spend a few seconds breathing deeply to center yourself. Breathe in the energy of the present moment. Exhale the energy of the past and any expectations of the future. Repeat this as many times as needed. You'll feel when you're ready to begin, because your entire body will be comfortable and relaxed.

- **When you're centered and present**, call on the energy of the circuit. First attune your mind to the circuit by saying, "I now attune myself to the energy of the *circuit name*." Then bring the energy to you by saying, "I call in the energy of the *circuit name*." Finally, circulate the energy in your body by repeating the circuit name three times. In the initial stages of training, doing this out loud will signal to your brain the specific energy vibration with which you want your body and brain to resonate.

- **Once you've practiced** and can confidently channel solar energy waves, you'll be able to simply think the phrase or imagine the circuit shape, and energy will respond immediately.

- **If you feel that your connection to a circuit** has been broken at any time, simply repeat the name of the circuit three times in order to reestablish the connection.

- **Any circuit can be used in any way**, on any part of the body. You can use one large circuit to encompass the entire body, or smaller circuits for targeted healing. I recommend that you start by using a single large circuit to attune the entire body to its frequency. As you master the circuits of a level, you can initiate many smaller circuits simultaneously in various parts of the body.

A FEW POINTERS

- **Generally speaking,** a clockwise circuit winds up and gathers energy as it breaks through and enters the body, while a counterclockwise circuit releases and relaxes energy, pulling it outside the body. These two work like yin and yang. When yin is optimized, it switches to yang. As your practice with solar energy circuits deepens, you will be able to use these complementary circuits at the same time.

- **You can direct the movement** of each circuit in a rapid motion or in a more gentle way depending on your purpose. If you want to relax a certain body part, you may use a circuit in a gentle fashion. If you want to release blockages or a stubborn emotional issue, you may imagine the circuit rotating very rapidly and powerfully.

- **Before calling on solar energy,** first determine where you will focus and what channel you will use to extract stagnant energy. Suppose your tongue is inflamed. You'll want to call on solar energy with your mind focused on your tongue, and extract stagnant energy through your mouth. All you have to do is let the energy flow out of your body, using any nearby channel.

- **If some part of your body** is uncomfortable or hurts, apply the circuit to that part. Focus on that area, calling in the circuit and moving it around and rotating it to purify the energy there.

LEVEL 1: CIRCUITS FOR CIRCULATION

While the four circuits in Level 1 have different individual attributes, they all function to release stagnant energy that may block a healthy flow of energy. These circuits are relatively gentle and fluid compared to the circuits in the other levels, and they're an essential first step because they prepare the body for more dynamic energy in future lessons. Like water flowing down a drain, they move in a gentle, circular motion.

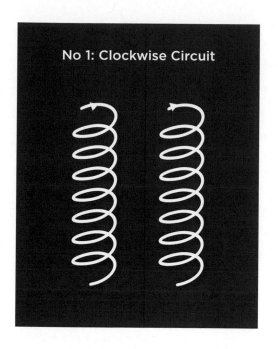

No 1: Clockwise Circuit

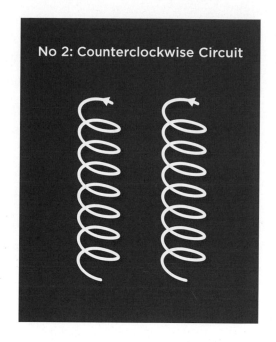

No 2: Counterclockwise Circuit

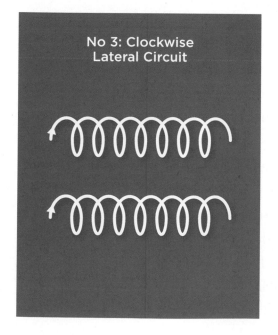

**No 3: Clockwise
Lateral Circuit**

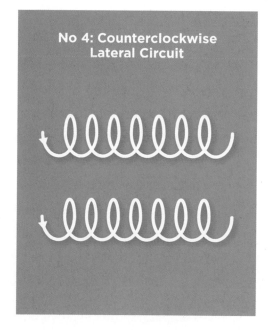

**No 4: Counterclockwise
Lateral Circuit**

LESSON 1: CLOCKWISE CIRCUIT

The Clockwise Circuit comes first because it prepares your body and mind by replacing old, stagnant energy with new, fresh energy. When blocked energy, unexpressed emotions, and repressed memories persist, your focus is fragmented. When your mind is tethered to the past or anxious about the future, you're less likely to be effective in the present.

Once you've received and filled your body and mind with this circuit's energy, the energy blockages will be naturally cleared, and you'll sink into the here and now. At this point, you'll begin to enhance your skills of intention, energy mastery, and manifestation. This circuit brings a healthy, unencumbered sense of well-being and peace.

USING THE CIRCUIT

Sit or lie in a comfortable position, making your back as straight as possible. Breathe in the present moment. Exhale the energy of the past and future. Repeat as needed. Once you are completely centered and present, speak aloud: "I now attune myself to the energy of the Clockwise Circuit."

Again speak aloud: "I call in the energy of the Clockwise Circuit." Depending on your sensitivity level, you may feel a shiver go through your spine or a tingling sensation on the top of your head when you initially connect to the circuit. If you're unpracticed, it's important not to be attached to any particular sensation. Any sensation, or no sensation at all, is OK—and part of your process. The more you practice, the more aware of the energy you'll

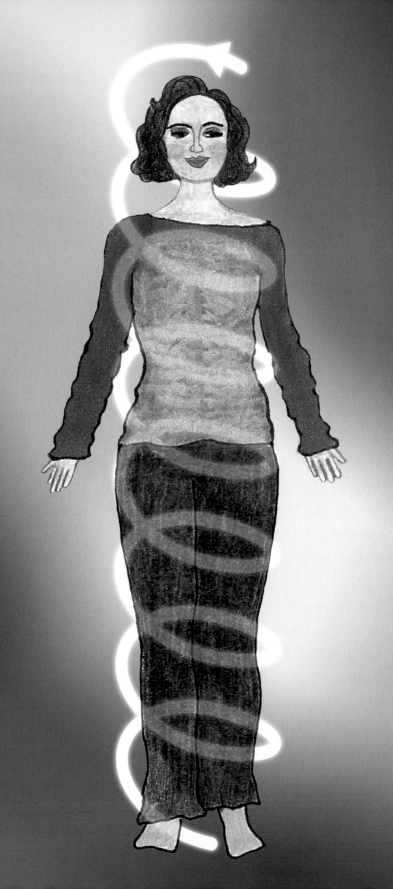

become. If you don't feel anything, don't be discouraged. Just keep practicing. Eventually your mind will quiet, your energy sense will open, and a whole new world of perception will be available to you.

When you've connected with the circuit, it's time to circulate the energy through your body. You can begin the energy flow by repeating the circuit name: "Clockwise Circuit, Clockwise Circuit, Clockwise Circuit." You'll begin to feel a sweeping circular sensation at the top of your head. Allow yourself to observe the sensation without any attachment.

In the beginning, don't try to move it, make it faster or more powerful, or augment or control the flow of energy in any way. Just notice the sensation as you allow the energy of the universe to move through you. You are working with solar energy at the universal level, and it flows of its own accord. Trying to control it with your mind may interrupt the flow. By opening yourself as a channel of these higher energies, you are agreeing to let them move through you, entrusting yourself to the flow of universal principles. After you are familiar with the energy flow of the circuit, you can proceed to direct the circuit's movements with the power of your mind.

Focusing on the crown of your head, you'll begin to feel the coiling circuit enter, winding clockwise. Immediately you will feel a release of tension in your head and a refreshing, cool sensation in your brain. You may hear audible creaks as the plates of your skull begin to move and release pressure; this is totally normal as your brain begins to regulate itself. Observe the energy circuit as it coils through your whole body, almost as if it were screwing itself into your body, gathering energy in one direction and properly centering your body. You'll notice that the energy circuit lets you enter a state free of thoughts and ideas. Any distracting thoughts will naturally be released as the energy in your mind flows harmoniously and unifies.

FOR THE REMAINING CIRCUITS

Now that you've familiarized yourself with the basic steps, you're ready to learn the remaining circuits. The instructions for Lessons 2 through 12 are a little less detailed, but you can review the process at any time by revisiting Lesson 1.

Remember the process of attunement, connecting, and channeling energy. For attunement, say out loud: "I now attune myself to the energy of the *circuit name*." For connecting, say out loud: "I call in the energy of *circuit name*." For channeling energy, repeat the circuit name three times or more.

Keep in mind the importance of your focus as you work with the circuits. Concentrate on the sensations in your body, and trust that the circuits are working. Note how each circuit affects you personally, and how its effects change over time. As they become familiar, direct the circuits with more specific intentions for your natural healing.

LESSON 2: COUNTERCLOCKWISE CIRCUIT

This next progression may feel a bit more powerful than the Clockwise Circuit. The energetic vortex created by this circuit moves through the whole body, gently releasing the stagnant energy and unresolved information within your body's cellular memory. If you have cold hands and feet, heavy limbs, congestion or tiredness in the chest, or if you fatigue easily, this circuit will raise your body temperature and open the circulation of energy throughout the body.

USING THE CIRCUIT

When you're completely relaxed and present, speak aloud: "I now attune myself to the energy of the Counterclockwise Circuit."

You'll begin to feel a change of sensation as your cells begin to resonate at the vibratory level of the circuit. Now say: "I call in the energy of the Counterclockwise Circuit." You'll feel warm energy skimming the surface of your crown. To draw this energy farther into your body, repeat the circuit name: "Counterclockwise Circuit, Counterclockwise Circuit, Counterclockwise Circuit."

Focusing your attention on the crown of your head, you'll feel the coiling circuit enter, winding counterclockwise. Immediately you will feel energy traveling through your body like a screw being unscrewed. Tension, stiffness, and stagnant energy will be pulled from your body. You may feel a sensation of heat or a subtle but quick vibration in areas that are releasing blockages. This circuit, while dynamic, has the attribute of complete balance, so it will always center your body.

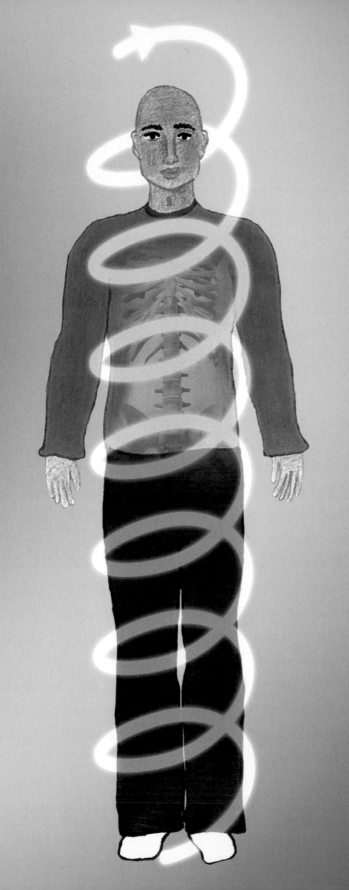

LESSON 3: CLOCKWISE LATERAL CIRCUIT

The Clockwise Lateral Circuit is a powerful tool for releasing emotional toxicity and negative memories bound to your body's energy system. You will discover that when negative memories are resolved, an associated tension in your body—conscious or unconscious—will also be released. After experiencing this circuit's energy, you'll feel more optimistic, hopeful, and excited about creating your life anew. Both Clockwise Lateral Circuit and Counterclockwise Lateral Circuit are especially effective for opening your heart and clearing emotional clutter.

USING THE CIRCUIT

After calling in the energy of the circuit and circulating it throughout your body, focus your attention on your chest. This circuit may enter from the front, back, left, or right. You'll feel a cool, refreshing energy swirling along the surface of your flesh that instantly warms as it enters. Your chest, lungs, and back will relax, and your breathing will become deep and effortless. If bad, unwanted memories arise, imagine hooking them to the ring of the continuously moving circuit and sending them flowing gently away. As you concentrate on the circuit, your mind's disordered tangle of thoughts will naturally harmonize, becoming organized and methodical, and you'll be able to focus on what you want to create in the here and now. The past will no longer affect what you desire, the choices you make, or the actions you take. You are free.

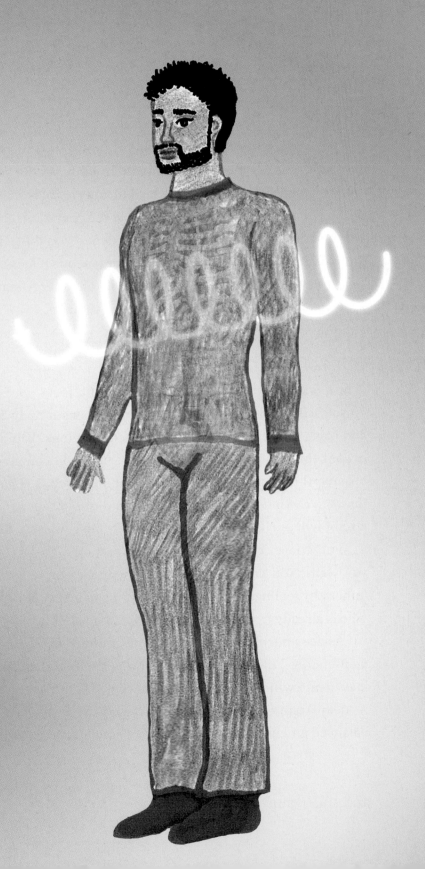

LESSON 4: COUNTERCLOCKWISE LATERAL CIRCUIT

The Counterclockwise Lateral Circuit will help you release the pent-up emotions more deeply and thoroughly. As the suppressed emotional energy that has been held in your body is released, you will feel a sudden decrease in physical and nervous tension. You will be amazed at how free and unburdened you'll feel by letting go. This circuit brings you a natural, spontaneous release, resulting in a stress-free mind and body. When the old energy leaves you, a spacious room for new energy to come in remains.

USING THE CIRCUIT

When you're completely relaxed and present, focus your attention on your chest. Rotating to the left as it enters your body from front and back, left and right, this circuit acts as a lens. You can watch distant things as if through a telescope, and you can magnify and observe things close up as if through a microscope. There are no limits to the lens of consciousness, and the solar energy from this circuit will purify whatever your lens of consciousness focuses on.

Pull the circuit to travel to the past, the future, wherever you want. You can savor beautiful memories or let go of bitter, unhealthy feelings from the past, or you can meet your future self, who is already living the life you've dreamed about, and get advice.

As deep purification happens, you naturally start exhaling stagnant energy. You may extend your arms and body, and your spine may create winding or squeezing movements as a healing process. As deep, trapped emotional blocks are released, you become more balanced and non-compulsive and feel unconditional happiness.

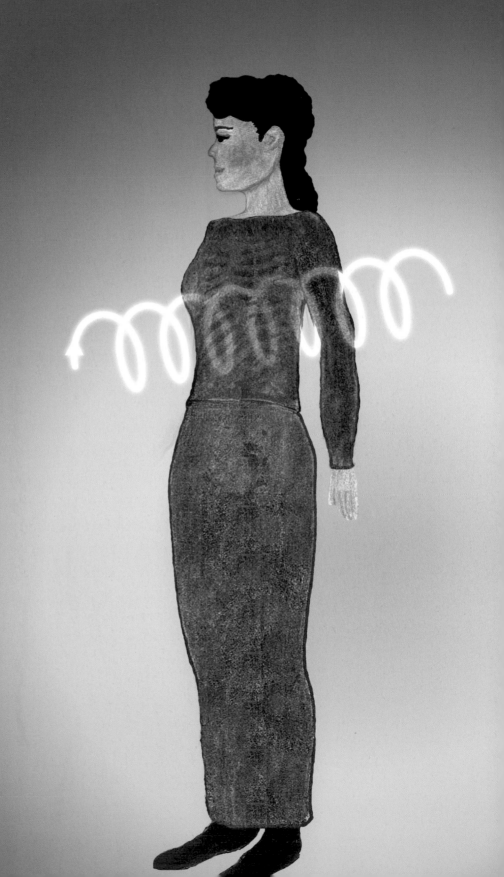

LEVEL 2:
CIRCUITS FOR POWER

The three circuits in Level 2 are empowering circuits. Now that you've removed the stagnant energy blockages and activated your body's energy system through the first level of training, the second level focuses on bringing power into the body, mind, and spirit.

You may notice from the circuit illustrations that the circuits in this level are a bit more electric, active, and dynamic. They bring those same qualities to your body's energy system. When you train with these three circuits, the sensations you experience are also likely to be electric, sizzling, and strong. The strength of these circuits allows you to dig deep into the crevices of stagnant energy in your body and pull out what you couldn't reach with the relatively gentle circuits in Level 1. Like flipping on a light switch, your energy will also be "turned on" and buzzing.

In giving you a new level of energy, these circuits also deepen your awareness and insight, providing you with a new and empowering perspective. The new lens through which you can see the world with these circuits frees you from any victim consciousness or other limiting beliefs that hamper your natural healing power.

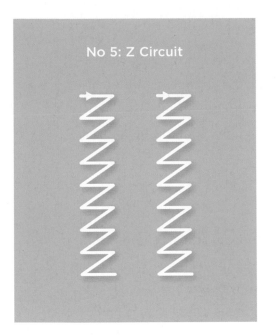

No 5: Z Circuit

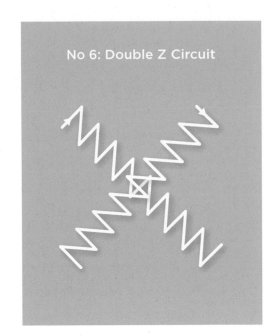

No 6: Double Z Circuit

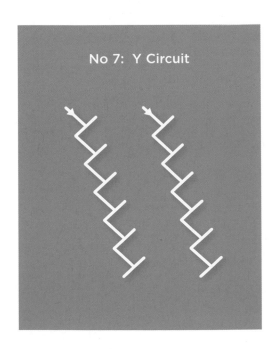

No 7: Y Circuit

LESSON 5: Z CIRCUIT

The Z Circuit is an activator that acts as an eraser. It scrubs the toxins and imbalance from your body, leaving you feeling physically healthy and vibrant. You'll feel more present and motivated, and you'll move through your daily life with more stamina and power.

USING THE CIRCUIT

As you call the energy of the Z Circuit to you and repeat its name, sense its dynamic energy buzzing through your body. The circuit will zoom into your body through the top of your head.

Imagine it disinfecting and normalizing every cell it passes. The energy wipes your body clean of damaged and unbalanced cells from head to toe, leaving your body feeling clean, clear, and warm. As unbalanced energy flow harmonizes into its natural state of balance, you'll feel your trunk properly aligning from front to back and side to side. Take a moment to enjoy the sense of well-being, and feel the activation of power and stamina in your vital, healthy body.

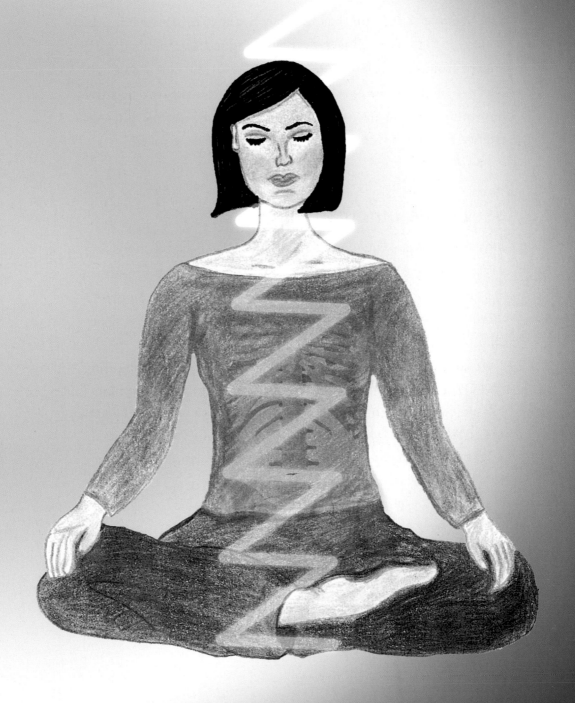

LESSON 6: DOUBLE Z CIRCUIT

The Double Z Circuit has similar healing properties to the Z Circuit, but its healing power is amplified by applying solar energy from two different directions. Stress and imbalance will dissipate as the solar energy from this circuit burns the negative imprints lingering in your body. This circuit restores physical vitality, emotional well-being, and a sense of passion for life.

USING THE CIRCUIT

This circuit enters your body like two crackling lightning bolts that strike diagonally across the center of your body. The Z Circuit from the previous training instantly warms the body, but the Double Z Circuit creates so much cellular vitality that you may notice a sensation of extreme heat.

Your whole body seems to float, like vapor rising from boiling water. All negative memories or feelings or unsolved problems will melt away. Stay immersed in this circuit for a while, and you'll find that the stiffness in your body has relaxed, your chest feels refreshed, and the feeling of constriction that was once there has been blasted away.

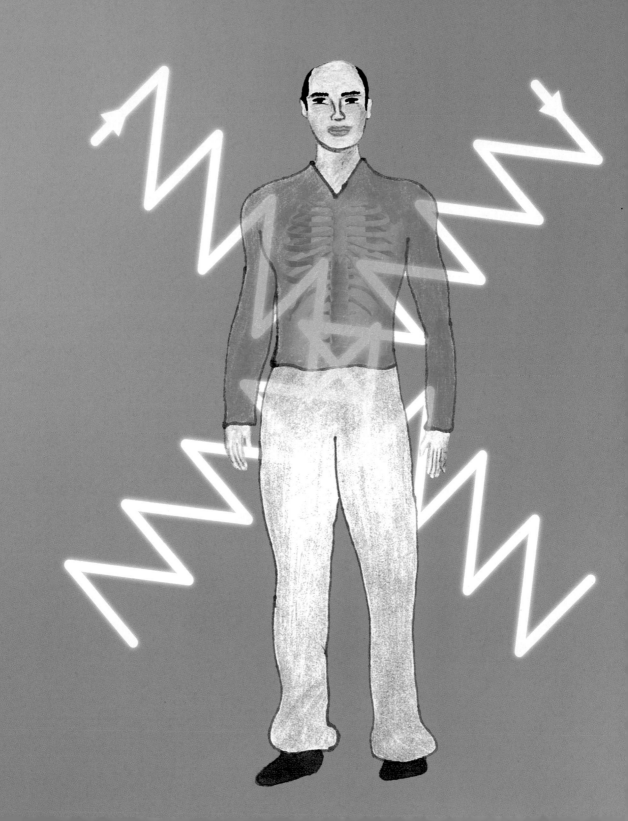

LESSON 7: Y CIRCUIT

The Y Circuit moves through every nook and cranny of your body, deep-cleaning away any emotional residue, pathogens, and energy blocks not cleared by the previous circuits. It works at a nano-level, reaching the corners of every cell and the spaces between cells. All residual darkness is replaced by the light of life, recalibrating your energy to a neutral state and preparing your template for optimal creation in future levels.

USING THE CIRCUIT

Like a sort of "darkness detector," the Y Circuit enters through the top of your head, infiltrating every nook and cranny of your body. For a more powerful experience you may call in the Z Circuit in conjunction with the Y Circuit and allow the two to move as one. When these two circuits enter at the same time, they'll clean every corner of your body because of their ability to reach deeply into the small and narrow places, leaving the purest light of life in their wake. You may notice a subtle vibration in places where you have abnormal symptoms, and you may feel a slight sting—as if unhealthy energy has been poked by an acupuncture needle—but you will also feel clean, clear, and refreshed.

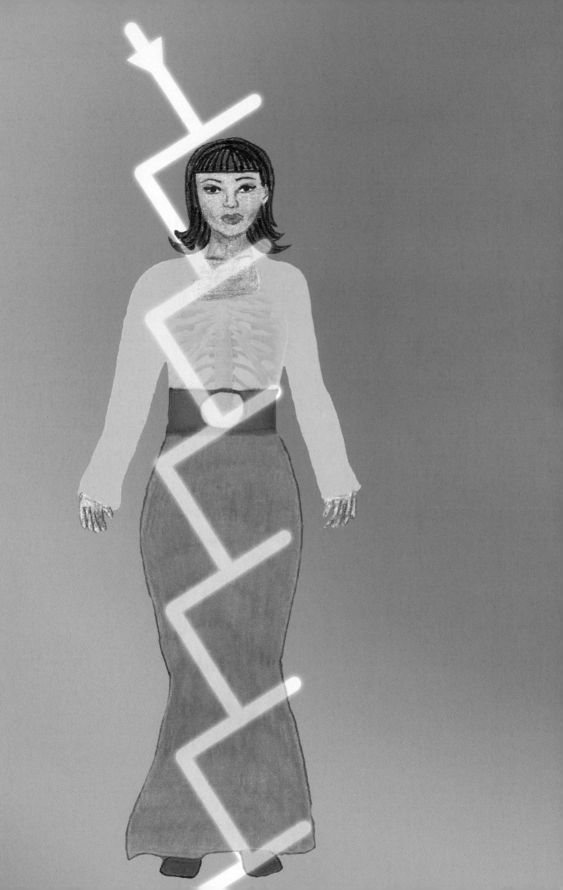

LEVEL 3: CIRCUITS FOR CREATION

The four circuits of Level 3 help you develop the ability to manifest health, happiness, and peace on your own by receiving and sending solar energy with the power of your mind to your desired results. As you progress through the circuits of Level 3, you'll be able to sense the subtle energetic changes inside and outside your body. Your awareness of your thoughts, emotions, and habits will increase, and you will experience enhanced focus.

Moreover, you will be able to change energy instantly from negativity to positivity as soon as you are aware of it. Conflict begins to resolve itself, and you'll feel happier and more whole. There's still some energetic cleaning in this phase of your training, and this will take place at a deeper level, so simply observe anything that comes up with complete openness and trust that it will be resolved once and for all.

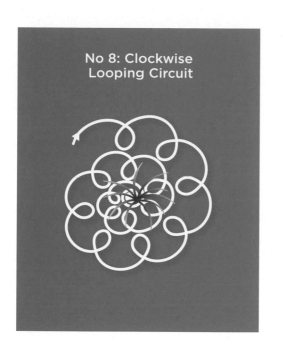

No 8: Clockwise Looping Circuit

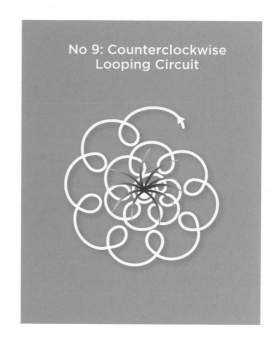

No 9: Counterclockwise Looping Circuit

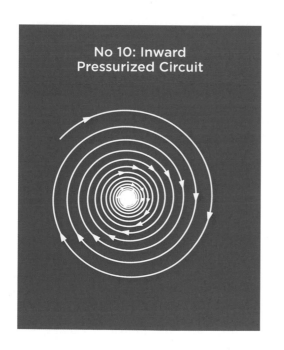

No 10: Inward Pressurized Circuit

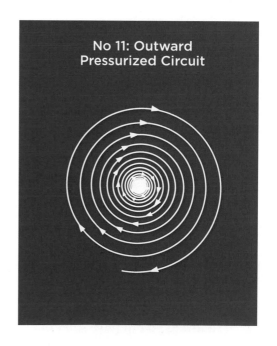

No 11: Outward Pressurized Circuit

LESSON 8: CLOCKWISE LOOPING CIRCUIT

The Clockwise Looping Circuit creates a tight and dynamic movement of energy that draws inward toward its center, strongly pulling all irregularities into its core—much like a black hole in space that pulls all neighboring stars and debris into its farthest point. The energy at the center of the Clockwise Looping Circuit compresses so tightly that all remaining unbalanced cells and probabilities for illnesses are burned by the hot pressure and intense heat at the core. Once this energy is transformed, you'll feel a great energetic explosion of heat and vibration billow outward from the core, like the birth of a new universe. This creates great and lasting power and vitality in the body.

USING THE CIRCUIT

After entering the body, the energy of the Clockwise Looping Circuit will circle in your chest from all directions. As the spirals rotate inward, moving fast, energy is drawn tightly into the core of the circuit. The more the energy collects, the more it is amplified. If you are physically unwell somewhere, focus on that area. Imagine the circuit surrounding any unbalanced cells, pulling them to the absolute center point. Observe all irregularities and darkness being melted by the intense heat. As the transformed and intensely bright energy is compressed and pressurized to the maximum, a great explosion of pure energy showers outward in all directions, bathing you in pure solar energy of light, vibration, and heat.

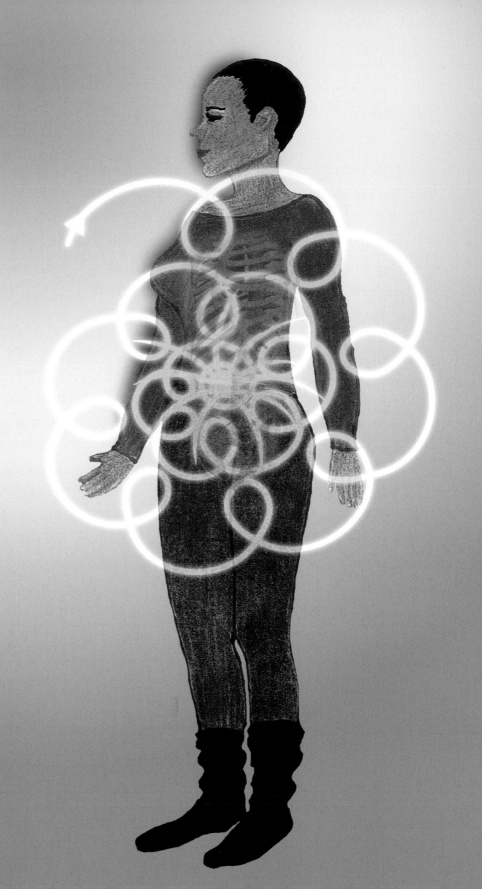

LESSON 9: COUNTERCLOCKWISE LOOPING CIRCUIT

Like the Clockwise Looping Circuit of the previous lesson, the Counterclockwise Looping Circuit rotates inward, moving toward the center. This circuit works like a vacuum cleaner, sucking up all residual ash left over from the previous circuit. The circuit ensures that a concentrated renewal of the body is maintained, removing any probability of dark energy manifesting itself.

USING THE CIRCUIT

Feel the Counterclockwise Looping Circuit circle in the space of your chest from all directions. As the spirals rotate inward, moving fast, any residual stagnant or cold energy left from the previous circuit is sucked into the core, like a powerful vacuum sucking up ash and debris.

Once the lifeless ash is received by the core of the circuit, it is transformed into pure particles of life that burst outward, surrounding your entire being with sparkling particles of potentiality.

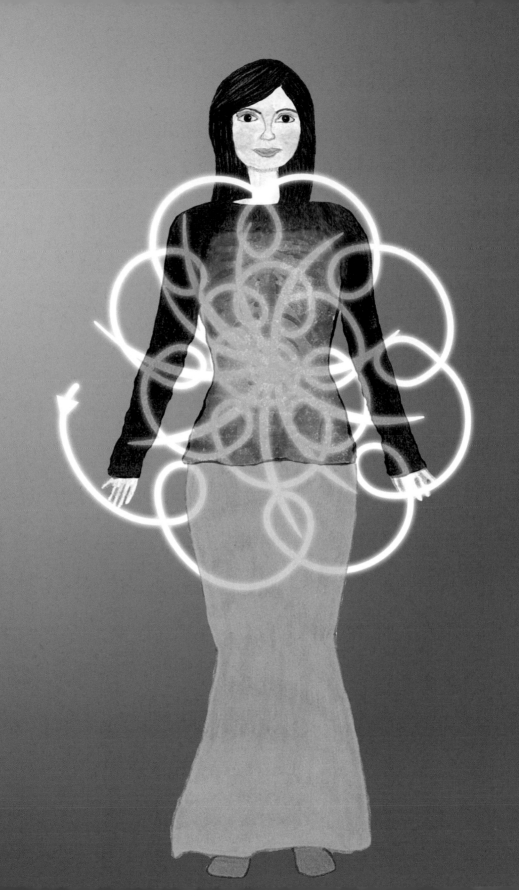

LESSON 10: INWARD PRESSURIZED CIRCUIT

The Clockwise Pressurized Circuit moves like a powerful hurricane. This inward, quick-moving circuit makes it impossible for your body to hold anything but the vibrant and vigorous light of life. It restores the gleam and vitality that is our original state of being and ensures optimal health of body, mind, and spirit.

USING THE CIRCUIT

Feel the intense power of the Inward Pressurized Circuit move through you like the most powerful hurricane. Imagine the circuit spinning unbalanced cells, surrounding them and applying pressure to each of them from the outside in.

The energy grows hot like a furnace and breaks the atomic bonds of matter, causing them to collapse and ensuring that they vanish before they have a chance to reproduce. In the end, only pure light—solar energy—remains.

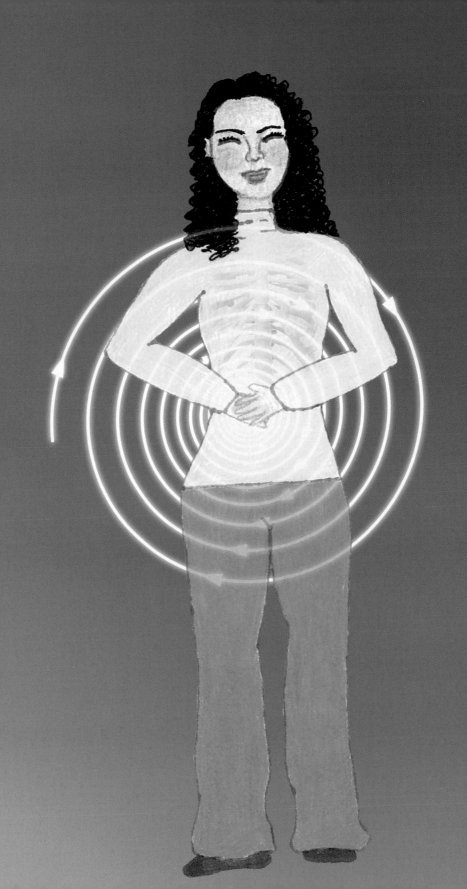

LESSON 11: OUTWARD PRESSURIZED CIRCUIT

The Outward Pressurized Circuit rotates outward from its center to infinity. This circuit works like a vacuum cleaner, sucking up any ash left from the previous circuit. This circuit is the tipping point, the light that pierces the darkness to infuse your energy field with the warm, bright solar energy of the sun.

USING THE CIRCUIT

This circuit moves delicately but quickly, in very fine lines like the growth rings of a tree. Feel the gentle squeeze of pressure created from the inside out, uprooting and expelling any pathogenic cells or any ash left from the previous circuit. Make use of the circuit's spiraling, rotating power, and you'll be able to break through any place your energy flow is blocked or stagnated.

You will refresh the energy field of every cell in your body as well as the collective energy fields surrounding your body. Imagine a pathway of light piercing the surrounding darkness and warm, bright solar energy pouring down on you from above.

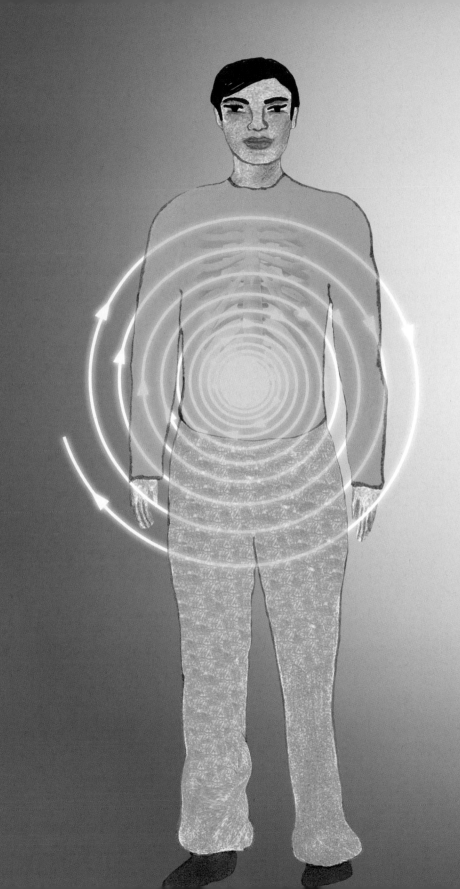

LEVEL 4:
CIRCUIT FOR COMPLETION—
MASTER CIRCUIT

An activated Solar Body is the optimal condition for living a healthy life full of abundant creation. A person with a vibrant Solar Body is not only nourished by their own light, but also nourishes their surroundings by the light that emanates from within. A person with a complete and full Solar Body is a blessing in the world and leaves their light-print everywhere they go. This master circuit contains all of the healing properties from the previous 11 circuits and makes them whole and intact. Healing happens effortlessly as the circuit manifests its completeness.

All of us and everything around us are made of elementary particles of energy. Not only is your body made of these particles, but so is your consciousness. I call these LifeParticles, the smallest unit comprising all life. These particles transmit the information that gives rise to the diverse phenomena of life. The LifeParticle Sun symbolizes the source of solar energy. It represents the purest, clearest energy, the source of love and creative power.

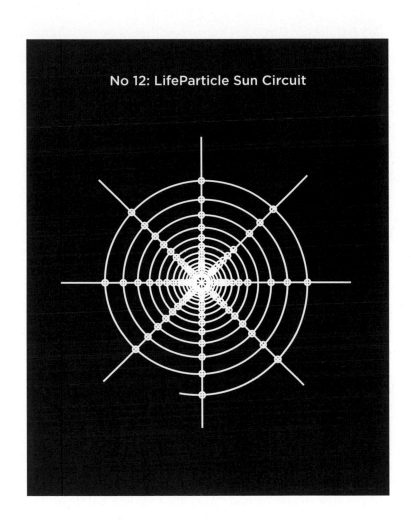

No 12: LifeParticle Sun Circuit

LESSON 12: LIFEPARTICLE SUN CIRCUIT

The LifeParticle Sun Circuit is the circuit that appears when you're in perfect sync with your natural healing power. Within a moment of encountering this circuit, the complete balance of Water-up, Fire-down is achieved. Your body is strong, your mind is at peace, and your spirit shines brightly. Health, peace, and joy well up automatically and naturally within you. This circuit will assist you in becoming an optimized human being.

USING THE CIRCUIT

Imagine the LifeParticle Sun Circuit surrounding you in all directions as all the molecules in your body recover their perfect balance and gleam with undiluted life energy. The temperature in your body rises and the warm fluid energy flows unencumbered throughout your body. Perfect harmony. Perfect balance. Perfect health. Your whole body is surrounded by solar energy LifeParticles. Energy rises through your chakra line and showers around you, surrounding you with a perfectly round, brilliant aura of solar energy—a balanced torus. Feelings of spiritual and cosmic rapture as well as physical ecstasy overtake you. Your soul shines brightly like the sun; your body is as light as a feather; and your convictions are as solid as diamonds.

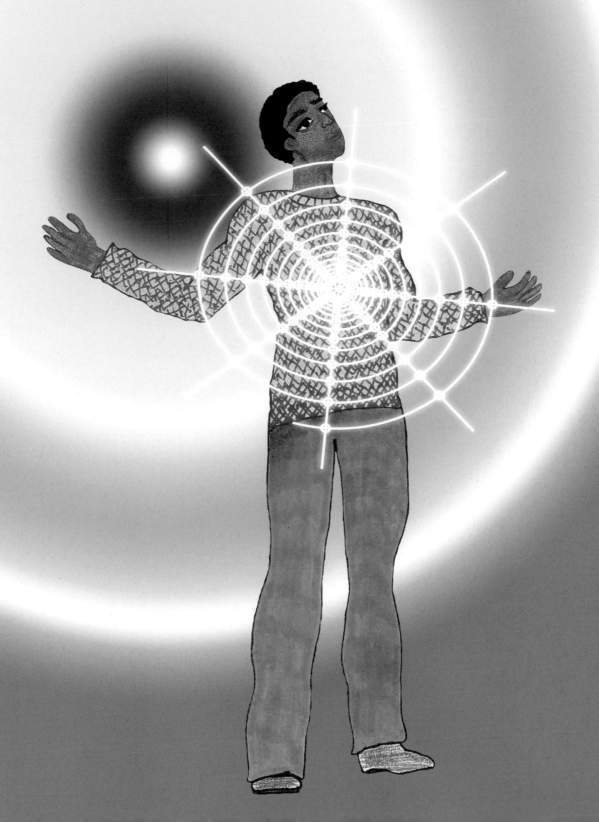

WORKING WITH THE
12 CIRCUITS ALL AT ONCE

You've learned how to work with each circuit and utilize its healing properties so far. Now that you are tuned to the subtle vibrations of every circuit, you can move on to receive the 12 circuits of solar energy all at once. All you have to do is entrust your body to the flow of energy with a pure and open heart. Just receive the solar energy pouring down on you from above and below, from left and right, from all directions. You can use this technique at any time that you want to uplift your energy and powerfully experience your connection to the limitless power within.

USING THE CIRCUIT

Sitting or lying in a comfortable position, breathe in the energy of the present. Exhale the energy of the past and the future. When you're completely relaxed and present, speak aloud: "I now attune myself to the energy of the 12 solar energy circuits."

You'll feel a change of sensation as your cells start to resonate at the vibratory level of the circuits. Now say: "I call in the energy of the 12 solar energy circuits." You'll feel the warm energy of the circuits skimming the surface of your crown. To draw this energy farther into your body, repeat aloud: "Solar energy circuits, solar energy circuits, solar energy circuits."

Within a minute, the 12 circuits will enter your body at the speed of light. They come from all directions, left and right, above

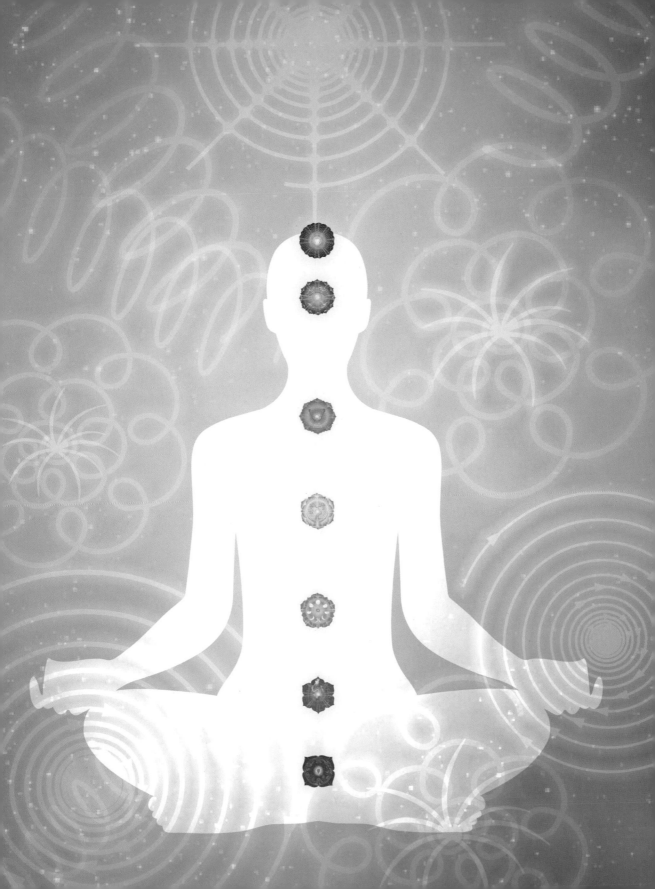

and below. All you have to do is open your mind and accept them. You don't need to try hard to remember the shape of each of the circuits, or to reproduce their movements in your brain. There's nothing that you have to do especially, and nothing you can do, either. Simply entrust yourself to the flow and accept the solar energy.

Small or large vibrations may happen throughout your body. Powerful, vigorous vibrations and body movements will gradually subdue, and you will become more relaxed and quiet. Your body may grow warmer, or as cold energy leaves, it may sting or feel colder. Your body will warm again once the cold energy exits. You may feel as if you are floating in water or through space, your whole body dissolving into the luminescent energy. You don't need to do anything besides maintaining the connection to the solar energy. Just receive, surrender, and let the solar energy move through you.

The solar energy knows what it's doing, expelling everything it should—toxins, pathogens, stagnant or cold energy imbalance, and negative memories. There is only one thing for you to do: open your mind and accept the solar energy, letting the perfect healing power within you handle everything by itself.

As you are transformed into a Solar Body and experience the magnificent beauty of your being, an earnest desire to help others and the world radiates with splendid luminescence. You can't help but choose the desire, because it springs from your purest essence, your original mind.

SOLAR BODY
EXERCISES

THREE MOVEMENTS FOR RESTORING HEALTH

Solar Body Exercises are a way to activate natural healing power by raising the body's temperature and optimizing its energy balance through simple physical movements. For the past 30 years, I have researched, developed, and taught methods for restoring health of body and mind and developing the brain's potential. What I introduce here as Solar Body Exercises are the movements that countless people have found to be the simplest and most effective.

Many people have shared that these exercises helped restore their bodies and minds to a healthy state. Major Korean television broadcasters have introduced the Solar Body Method to a wide audience, and it has gained popularity in a short period of time through the media. There are good reasons for this. First, these exercises are so simple that it takes just a few minutes to learn them, yet the effects are outstanding. And you can do them anywhere and at any time. Of course, still another reason is that it costs nothing to learn the Solar Body Exercises.

Three exercises are included in the Solar Body Method:

- **Plate Balancing** involves rotating the arms in movements that are as natural as flowing water. This opens the whole body so that blood and energy flow to every nook and cranny. It trains muscles and joints, strengthens the energy center in the lower abdomen, and increases concentration through the sense of balance.

- **Toe Tapping** strengthens the lower body, improves agility, and releases energy massed toward the head due to stress so it can flow toward the lower body. It evenly stimulates the reaction points in the feet, improving bodily functions overall.

- **Brain Wave Vibration** relaxes the first cervical vertebra and medulla oblongata, where physical tension due to stress begins. Blood flow to the brain improves, and the temperature of the belly is raised to create the ideal temperature balance: cool head, warm lower abdomen.

Doing just these three things facilitates energy and blood circulation and causes body temperature to rise, producing what I call a Solar Body state. While all three exercises stimulate overall energy and blood circulation, Plate Balancing especially impacts the upper body, shoulders, and arms. Toe Tapping powerfully affects the lower body, hips, and legs, and Brain Wave Vibration targets the abdomen, spine, neck, and brain. Combining these three results in a completely holistic, full-body exercise.

It's good to do the exercises often, but even 10 minutes each for a total of 30 minutes every day is sufficient to sustain a Solar Body state. So I call these the 10-10-10 Exercise—three movements performed for 10 minutes each.

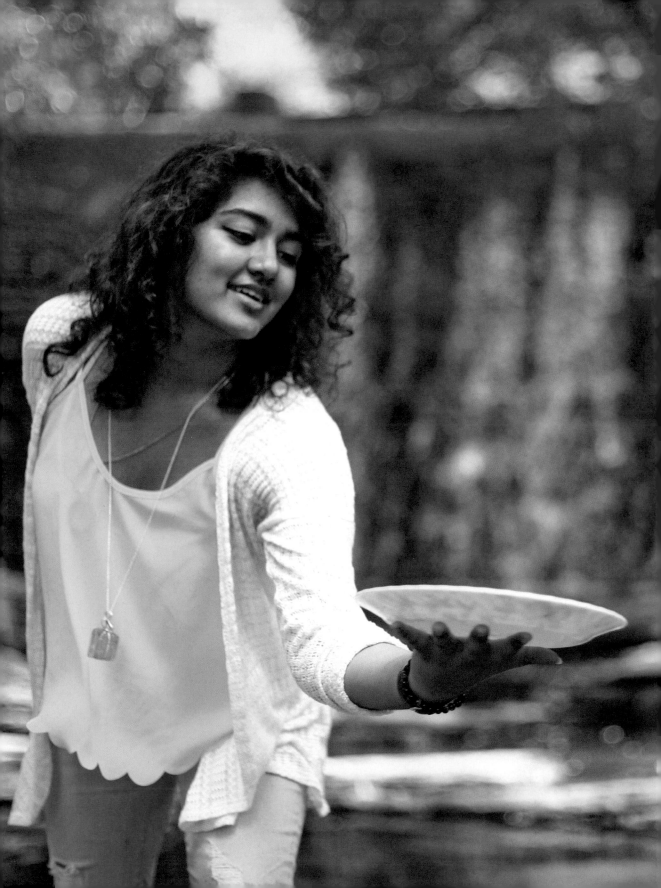

PLATE BALANCING

Plate Balancing involves moving your arm in a figure-eight pattern—a vertical infinity—while balancing a plate on your hand. This exercise strengthens the body's major joints and meridians (energy channels), especially the upper body and abdominal area.

You can use any kind of plate that fits comfortably in your hand, but you may want to use one that's not breakable, such as a plastic or heavy paper plate. You can also do the exercise without the plate, though balancing a plate requires greater concentration. Or you can use a book or other object instead. It's a good idea to use a plate until you can easily follow the exercise. After that you may do the exercise without a plate.

The following directions might feel a little involved at first, but you'll find the actual movement to be very simple.

Learn from a video online at SolarBodyMethod.com.

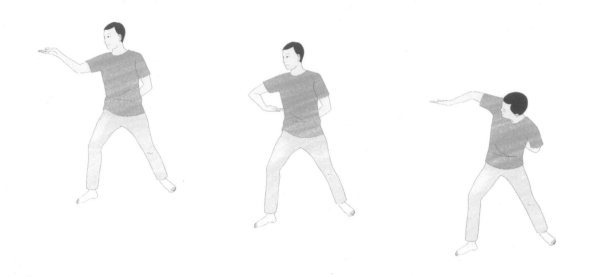

PLATE BALANCING WITH ONE HAND

1. Plant your right foot forward, about one and a half times your shoulder width from the other foot, with your toes pointing forward. Turn the left foot outward at about a 45-degree angle. Bend your knees slightly. Your stance should feel comfortable, balanced, and natural.

2. Balance a plate on the palm of your right hand and hold it at elbow height over your right knee. Rest the back of your left hand against your lower back. (If you don't have a plate, imagine that there's one.)

3. While leaning your upper body forward, pull your right hand (with the plate) in toward your body in a counterclockwise circle, pivoting around your elbow until your arm is straight

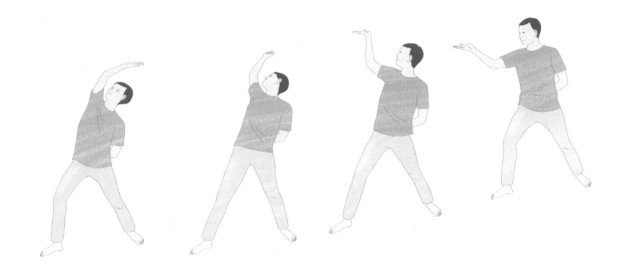

out to the side and twisted so that your palm is still facing upward. Then continue the circle with your elbow straight by moving your shoulder until your arm is extended in front of you. Remember to keep your palm facing upward throughout the motion.

4. Begin the second circle of the figure eight by moving your arm counterclockwise over your head as you extend your upper body back as far as you can. Look back at your hand as it circles behind you. Bend your elbow as much as you need to in order to keep your palm (and your plate) facing upward. As your hand passes behind you and comes around to its original position in front of you, straighten your upper body.

5. Repeat this spiraling, figure-eight motion several times. Then reverse the position of your body and do the same thing using the left hand.

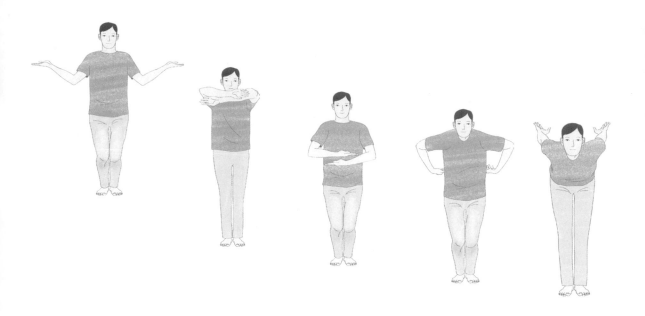

PLATE BALANCING WITH BOTH HANDS

1. Standing with your feet together and your palms facing
    upward, hold your hands comfortably at your sides. If you
    have trouble keeping your balance in this position, place your
    feet about a shoulder width apart. You can balance plates on
    your palms, or you may choose not to use them. You can also
    hold the plates in place with your thumbs.

2. Bend your upper body forward, bringing your hips back and
    using your lower back strength to keep your balance as you
    straighten your knees as much as you can. Keeping your knees
    straight will provide the most benefit to your back and legs.

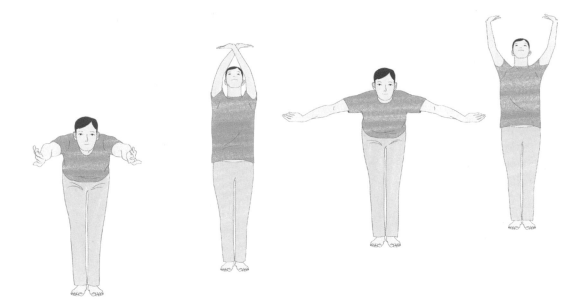

However, if you have trouble balancing in this position, you can bend your knees instead. As you bend forward, slowly pull your hands toward the side of your body and pivot them around your elbows until your arms are out to the side. Then with your palms facing upward, extend your arms out in front of you.

3. Raise your upper body, crossing your arms in front of you. Leaning your upper body backward, move each hand above your head in the biggest circle you can make. Then bring your hands back to their original positions Repeat this figure-eight movement.

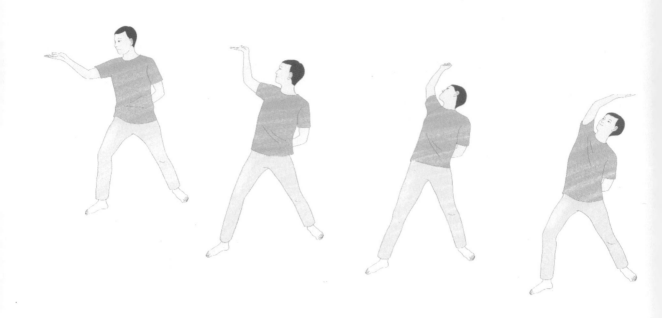

VARIATIONS: REVERSE PLATE BALANCING

Performing movements that you're not used to provides fresh stimulation for your brain. By making the figure eight in the opposite direction, and from top to bottom instead of bottom to top, you can stimulate a part of the brain that you haven't been using. This helps improve your ability to move your body with intention, and it helps you maintain the youthfulness and vitality of your brain.

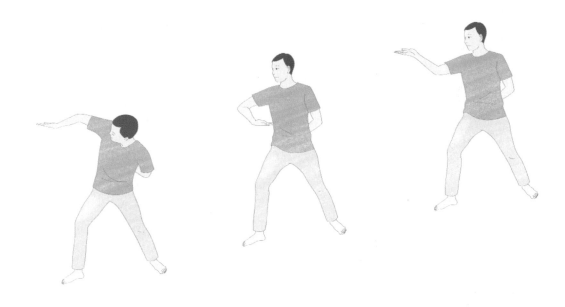

REVERSE PLATE BALANCING
WITH ONE HAND

1. With the palm facing up, hold your hand at head level and as far back as you can reach. Then move your hand clockwise toward your head and around in a large circle.

2. With your palm facing away from your body, bring your arm downward and make a smaller circle by the side of your body, pivoting your hand around your elbow.

3. Bring your hand back above your head again and repeat the spiraling, figure-eight motion.

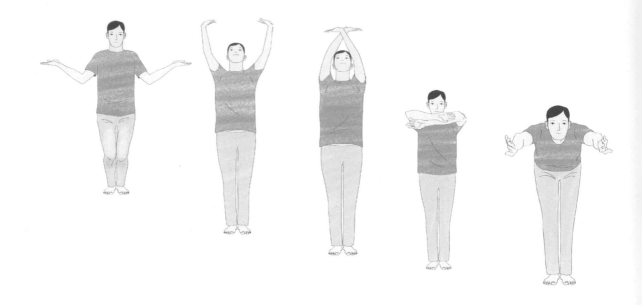

REVERSE PLATE BALANCING
WITH BOTH HANDS

1. With palms up, hold your hands at waist level. Open your
    arms out to the sides and bring them up and as far behind you
    as you can. Lean your upper body back and look at your hands.

2. Pivoting your hands around your elbows, cross your arms and
    lower them, bending forward at the waist at the same time. As
    your waist comes to a ninety-degree bend, uncross your arms
    and stretch them in front of you. This is one circle.

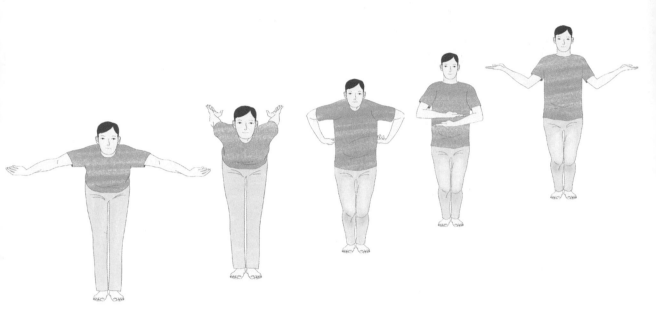

3. Keeping your palms facing upward, bring your straight arms out to the side until they are all the way behind you.

4. Bend your knees and raise your upper body as you pull your arms forward along your waist, keeping your palms up.

5. Cross your arms in front of your body and return to the original position. This completes the second circle of the figure eight.

6. You can repeat this movement as many times as you want to stretch both your body and brain.

WHY PLATE BALANCING
WORKS

Plate Balancing is super easy—all you have to do is keep moving your hands around in a figure eight. So how were so many people able to experience such incredible effects from such a simple exercise? A Korean woman named Hye-young Shin, for example, dropped 20 pounds and found relief from her chronic rheumatoid arthritis by practicing this exercise every day.

Allow me now to introduce the energy principles hidden in Plate Balancing. By experiencing them for yourself, I'm sure you'll come to realize that you can get a great workout for your entire body with this one exercise.

 Plate Balancing moves energy in a vortex.

Repetition of the simple arm movement in itself releases tension from the shoulders and arms. But it's much more effective if you feel energy—the life force that's in everything—while you're doing Plate Balancing. Here's how to do that.

Focus your mind on your upward-facing hand and imagine that a heavy pillar of energy is coming down toward your hand. Focus your mind on your palm. Imagine that the energy coming in through your palm flows along your arm through your elbow, shoulder, and torso, and is connected through your leg all the way to the bottom of your foot, forming an energy line in that side of your body. Now slowly perform the spiraling figure-eight motion, being careful not to scatter or disperse the weighty feeling of energy on your palm.

Now if you imagine that energy is coming up from the sole of the same foot and passing through that side of your body to move your arm around automatically, you'll be able to do the exercise more easily. The motion will take on its own tempo and become more dynamic. The circle above your head is naturally slow, and then your arm comes down quickly. When you follow the energy as the movement alternates between fast and slow, the overall motion picks up momentum.

This will be even more effective if you bend your knees slightly and rotate your hips. When you make the lower circle with your hand, press your hips toward the same side as the moving hand and circle them toward the front, following the motion of your hand. Continue the circle with your hips as you make the upper circle with your hand, pressing your hips to the other side and moving them around to the back. As you imagine energy coming up and rotating your waist and arms, follow the energy vortex and repeat the movement.

A vortex refers to a whirling, spiraling motion around a central axis. From the double helix of DNA to the movement of the Milky Way galaxy, the vortex represents nature's vital phenomena. When you practice Plate Balancing with body and mind in a state of relaxation and imagine the earth's vortex energy coming up through your feet to rotate your waist and arms, you can feel that energy being circulated in a powerful way. As you keep following this vortex movement of nature, the process of natural healing will begin in your body.

 ## *Plate Balancing opens up the major joints and Energy Channels.*

According to Eastern medicine, 12 major meridians or energy channels flow through the body and govern the internal organs. Six of these pathways go from the torso through the arms (lung, large intestine, pericardium, triple energizer, heart, small intestine meridians). The other six extend from the torso through the legs (stomach, spleen, bladder, kidneys, gallbladder, liver meridians). The reason Plate Balancing is so effective without straining the body, compared to other exercises, is that it opens up these meridians and the six major joints to promote circulation of blood and energy.

Not only do the circular arm motions of Plate Balancing stimulate the meridians through the arms, but the repetitive bending of the knees and the rotation of the waist stimulate the meridians of the legs. Doing Plate Balancing with both hands especially promotes blood and energy circulation throughout the entire body.

Along the pathways where these 12 meridians flow are about 365 energy points that act as stations where energy collects or goes in and out of the body. These are concentrated around the joints, the six major joints being the wrists, elbows, shoulders, hip joints, knees, and ankles. It's easy for murky, damp, or cold energy to stagnate at these joints. Not only is this congested energy conducive to infection, since it blocks energy flow, but it also makes your body feel heavy and lethargic. Repeatedly rotating and moving the joints for Plate Balancing is superbly effective at forcing out the congested energy, loosening both the joints and the surrounding stiff muscles.

When you start practicing Plate Balancing, your shoulders will probably be the first place to feel the impact. You'll feel how much tension and stiffness you had—not only in your shoulder joints but also in the muscles around them, including your trapezius and deltoid muscles and your triceps. To release this tension, it's important to perform the Plate Balancing exercise accurately. Moving your arms around without moving your shoulders isn't very effective. Work all the muscles of the chest and upper back by moving the shoulder area as much as you can when you rotate your arms. Do it this way, even for just a few days, and you'll feel much of the tension being released. Your shoulders will feel lighter.

As your shoulders start to loosen up, you'll be able to lean your upper body back farther and make bigger movements with your shoulders. You'll feel the stimulation concentrated along the side of the rib cage and the side muscles of the waist. You'll feel a stretch there when you bring your arm up after making the lower circle. It feels great—you can even feel it working on any excess flab.

Especially when doing Plate Balancing with both hands, bringing your hips back and bending your upper body forward with knees straight effectively stretches the bladder meridian along the back of the body. For the greatest impact, hold this posture for a bit. This gives your bladder meridian, which has a major influence on the flow of energy, a wonderfully refreshing stretch.

Making the circle above your head and leaning your upper body back stretches the stomach, spleen, and liver meridians along the front of the body. All six meridians in the legs can be worked more effectively if you lift up your big toes while doing Plate Balancing with both hands. That makes you use more leg strength to keep your balance.

 ### Plate Balancing strengthens the body's core.

It's easy to think of Plate Balancing as simply rotating the arms, but the more you practice it, the more you can feel that it's an excellent way to strengthen the lower back, lower belly, and hip joints that form your body's core.

When you make the large arm movements above your head, the pressure on your lower belly is increased through the process of maintaining your balance. You're working not only the transverse abdominals, the erector spinae muscles (which keep the spine erect), and the muscles of the pelvic area, but also the femoral muscles in the legs. Especially when you use both hands for Plate Balancing, repeatedly bending your upper body forward and then leaning backward improves lower back flexibility and increases abdominal strength.

To strengthen your core muscles even more effectively, place your feet farther apart when doing Plate Balancing with one hand, and bend your knees more deeply. As you make large rotations with your arms and shoulders, lean your upper body as far back as you can. The bigger you can make the rotational radius of your upper body and arms, the more strength your lower body and abdominal area will have to exert to maintain your body's balance.

Muscle elasticity increases through the repetition of these slow, low-intensity movements, and the muscles are strengthened by being supplied with energy. Plate Balancing is an outstanding core-strengthening exercise that effectively trains the muscles of the legs, pelvis, lower abdomen, and spine—without requiring you to struggle and sweat.

4 *Plate Balancing facilitates deep breathing naturally.*

It's perfectly OK to practice Plate Balancing without paying special attention to your breathing, but to experience greater aerobic benefits, it's even better to combine the movement with deep breathing.

Simply breathe in when you're moving your arm up and making a circle above your head, then breathe out as you bring your arm down and make a circle by the side of your body. When you lean your upper body back as your arm goes up, your rib cage and abdominal area expand as they're stretched vertically. Breathe as deeply as you can into that expanded space, and you'll feel your breath going into your chest and lungs and all the way to your lower belly. Breathe in while you slowly make the upper rotation, then start breathing out as you lower your arm. Continue exhaling as you make the lower circle and bend your upper body forward. You'll be able to feel fresh air being drawn into your body and stagnant energy being expelled, making your chest feel refreshed and your body lighter.

5 *Plate Balancing restores the balance of the autonomic nervous system.*

All the organs in our bodies are controlled by the autonomic nervous system that branches out from the spinal cord. But if balance is lost in the spine, which envelops the spinal cord, the increased burden on the surrounding muscles, tendons, and ligaments causes tension and adhesion. This adds pressure to the sympathetic nervous system, decreasing effective functioning of the organs it regulates—including the heart, lungs, and stomach.

Bending the upper body forward and backward and rotating the waist during Plate Balancing are highly effective for exercising the spine. You relieve energy stagnation and strengthen the erector spinae muscles that hold the spine erect. These movements also help correct misalignment of the spine and pelvis. When energy and blood circulation becomes fluid and the lower belly is strengthened this way, the sympathetic nervous system operates smoothly and balance is restored in the autonomic nervous system.

PLATE BALANCING
Q&A

Making the movements of Plate Balancing as big as possible is for those who have a basic level of good health. If physical restrictions prevent you from making large movements, keep the following guidelines in mind. Increase the flexibility of your body and your body temperature through simple stretching warm-ups prior to practicing Plate Balancing.

Q *What if I have trouble keeping my balance during Plate Balancing?*

A Because you shift your center of balance during Plate Balancing, you can lose your balance and fall if you have a weak lower body. Don't put your feet too far apart at first, don't lean back, and make only small circles with your hands until you become more used to the exercise. If this is difficult, support yourself by placing one hand against a wall, or sit in a chair and perform only the arm movement. With consistent practice, your legs and lower back will gradually develop strength, your joints will move more smoothly, and you'll be able to increase the effectiveness of the exercise.

Q *How many Plate Balancing repetitions should I do?*

A Do what's right for the condition of your body, but basically I recommend starting with a set of 10 repetitions using the right arm, 10 with the left arm, and 10 with both arms. Doing too many at the start could overexert your shoulders or arms. Take your physical condition into consideration before doing more, give yourself some time between sets, and add just one set at a time.

Once you develop some proficiency, increase the number of repetitions in a set by 10 to 20 and do one or two sets at a time. As your flexibility improves, you can do up to 30 reps and increase the number of sets. If your body is weak, doing more than 30 reps on one side may cause dizziness, so stick to a number that doesn't overextend your body. To maintain balance, do the same number on both sides. However, if there's greater tension in one shoulder, it's good to do more on that side.

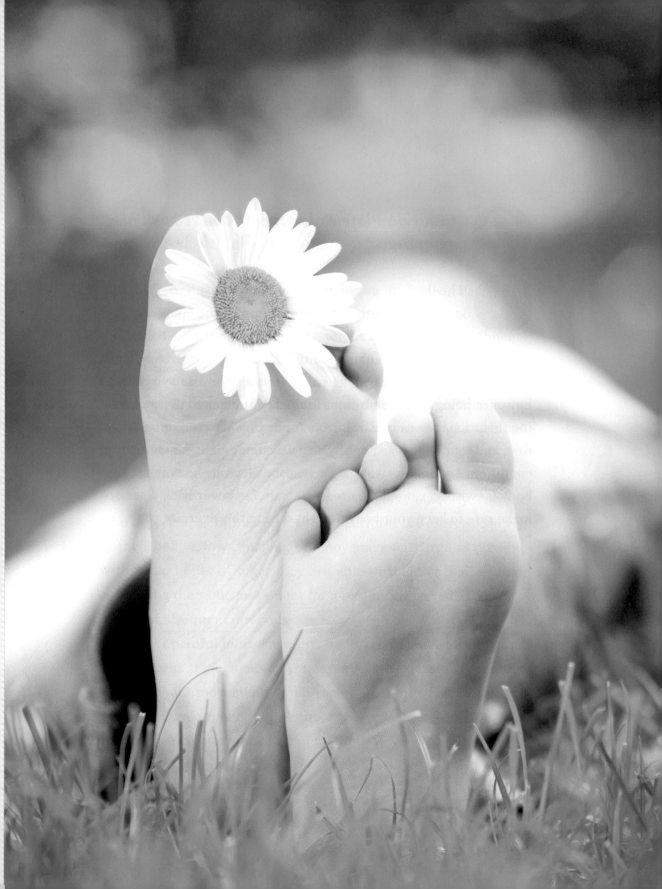

TOE TAPPING

An incomparable exercise for relaxing both the body and the mind, Toe Tapping consists of repeatedly hitting the inside edges of the feet together. This movement enhances the energy circulation of the six meridians flowing through the lower body. It also brings blood and energy from the upper body down into the lower body, cooling the head and warming the abdomen and lower body to create the optimal state of Water-up, Fire-down.

Many people who were bothered by leg pain before starting the Solar Body Exercises have shared that their joint pain has decreased from consistently practicing Toe Tapping. Their legs feel lighter when they walk, too.

Toe Tapping can be done sitting or lying down, but it's the most effective when done lying down. That opens up the hip joints.

Learn by watching a video online at SolarBodyMethod.com.

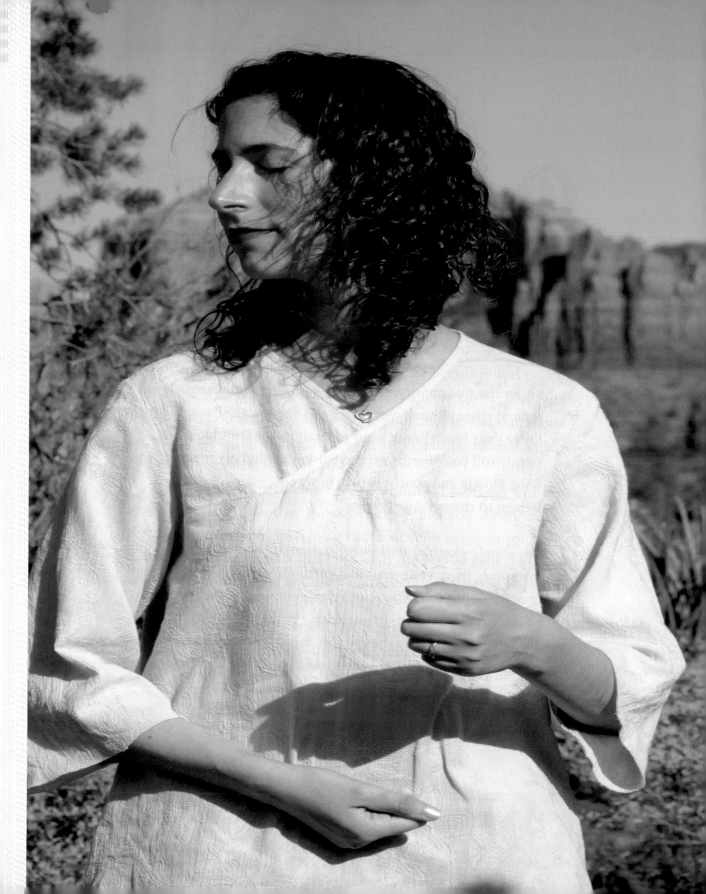

BRAIN WAVE VIBRATION

Brain Wave Vibration, the third movement in the Solar Body Exercises, is an effective way to quiet thoughts and emotions and to strengthen energy and blood circulation in the spine and lower abdomen, as well as the brain.

There's a behavioral pattern that's common when people want to stop thoughts from arising in their heads: they shake their head quickly from side to side. This isn't something that anyone has taught them. It happens automatically, like yawning or stretching, and within this natural occurrence is a natural healing method. Brain Wave Vibration was created to manifest this healing in a focused way.

To do Brain Wave Vibration, you can be seated in a chair or sit on the floor in a half-lotus posture. To strengthen your concentration, listen to percussion music made up of simple beats.

To watch an online video, go to SolarBodyMethod.com.

HOW TO DO
BRAIN WAVE VIBRATION

1. Straighten your lower back, comfortably relax your chest and shoulders, and rest your hands on your knees, palms up. Gently close your eyes and pull your chin in slightly so that your spine and head are aligned.

2. Mentally feel the inside of your body, going from your head to your neck and down along your spine. Move your consciousness slowly from the top of your body downward, as if doing a scan. When you reach your lower abdomen, concentrate your awareness there.

3. Make loose fists and gently tap your lower abdomen with your fists, palms up, alternating between left and right hands. You want to tap 2 inches below your navel. This is your body's energy center, and tapping strengthens the energy of this spot and makes it warmer.

4. As you continue to tap your lower abdomen, move your head, spine, and upper body to a natural rhythm. You'll get the feeling that you're pounding a drum to some beat, and you'll sense an inner rhythm and excitement rising up.

5. When your movements become rhythmic, begin shaking your head gently from side to side. Without moving too forcefully or

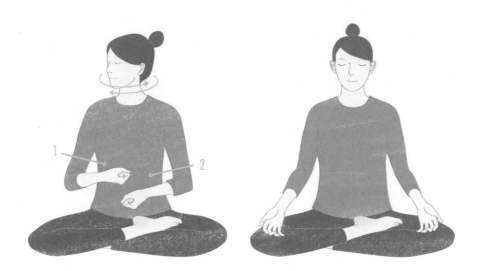

rapidly, try to feel your central axis. That's where your spinal cord passes and the center of your autonomic nervous system is located. Starting there, let go of the tension from your neck to your shoulders through the movement of gently shaking your head. Shake slowly at first, then a little faster once you're comfortable with the exercise. Don't think about anything at all. Simply shaking your head, imagining that you're shaking out all your thoughts, is the point of Brain Wave Vibration. If you feel any weariness or hot energy in your head, keep breathing it out through your mouth.

6. Continue exhaling through your mouth. Feel your breathing becoming lighter and more natural as the blockages in your chest open up and tension is released through your exhalations.

7. Once your lower abdomen feels somewhat warmer, use the palms of your hands to pat places in your body that seem to have blockages, opening the meridian points. If you have a stifling feeling in your chest, pat your chest. If your legs don't feel good, pat your legs. When the senses of your body have been revived, your hands will automatically go to the places that hurt.

8. Try this exercise for five minutes in the beginning and gradually increase to 30 minutes.

PRECAUTIONS FOR BRAIN WAVE VIBRATION

Brain Wave Vibration is so simple that it can be done by anyone of any age in just about any condition. However, like any exercise, you should not push yourself beyond your limits, and you should discuss your plans with your physician if you are concerned at all about your physical readiness to participate. Here are some precautions to keep in mind:

- **If you are very weak or too tense:** Before starting Brain Wave Vibration practice, relax your body by slowly turning your head left and right and rotating the shoulders forward and back. You can also do a few stretching exercises before you begin. If you stand during practice, make sure your feet are planted solidly on the ground.

- **If you cannot breathe well:** One good way to help your breathing is tapping your chest area with loose fists. This exercise helps release tension from the chest area, which is usually hard to stretch completely through ordinary stretching exercises. It is a good choice when you feel burdened by emotions because it works to open up the chest, which is where we tend to hold emotions like sadness and disappointment. You will feel a subtle vibration that spreads out from the chest to the whole body.

  When you first begin this exercise you may feel some pain in the chest area, which indicates that you have some blockage. If the pain is extremely severe, you should stop, but otherwise it is best to power through the pain to help open the blockage. As you exhale, make a long "ahhh" sound while patting your chest area. Focus on exhaling all air out of the lungs.

WHY BRAIN WAVE VIBRATION
WORKS

 Brain Wave Vibration calms your mind.

The simple motion of continuously shaking your head from side to side quiets the busy thoughts and emotions running amok in your brain. You naturally move your head this way when you want to stop the thoughts in your mind.

Try it yourself right now. Quickly shake your head from side to side for 10 seconds. Do thoughts keep coming up in your head, or do they diminish? Shake for a while, and you'll feel busy thoughts disappearing and your head becoming clearer. Once you understand this, you'll see that even the head-banging done by young people as they dance, or by members of rock bands, is really just an effective way to get rid of the tangle of thoughts afflicting them.

You can see this effect in the changing of brain waves that results from practicing Brain Wave Vibration. The sum of the brain's electrical activity can be measured as waves emanating from your head. Different wave frequencies indicate different states of consciousness. The brain waves that ordinarily appear when a person is engaged in daily activities are rapidly moving beta waves, which have a wavelength of 13 to 30 Hz (cycles per second). These are concentrated at the front part of the head when we talk, when we engage in conscious movement, when we're tense or excited, when we engage in complex thinking, and when we're worried. If mind and body relax and grow more comfortable, on the other hand, slower alpha waves (8 to 12 Hz) appear at the top and back of the head.

A study by the Korea Institute of Brain Science (KIBS) showed that Brain Wave Vibration often causes the brain to generate alpha waves, indicating that it is in a relaxed and calm state. Professor Hideo Arita of Japan's Toho University also found that brain waves after Brain Wave Vibration resemble the alpha state. Brain blood flow increased in the subjects of his study as well, and their entire brains were activated. There was also a marked decrease in indicators of tension, uneasiness, and fatigue, and in the psychological indicators of nervousness and feelings of awkwardness.

When busy thoughts won't stop coming, when your head feels heavy and hot, when you want to recover focus, try simply shaking your brain from side to side while tapping your lower abdomen with loose fists. You'll find that the simple movement of Brain Wave Vibration is amazingly powerful for making your brain free of distractions.

2. Brain Wave Vibration provides autonomic balance.

When we're stressed for long periods of time, the give-and-take between the sympathetic and parasympathetic nervous systems is out of balance. However, the simple movement of shaking your head from side to side is a superb way to relax and rebalance it. When we're under a lot of stress, we often feel tension in our shoulders and the back of the neck. When you've experienced this, have you ever massaged the back of your neck with your hand, or moved your head from side to side to release the tension? Everyone does these things naturally.

The neck and the back of the head are the first areas to tense up as blood surges toward the head when we're under stress. The concave point below the back of the head, where the skull and cervical vertebrae meet, is especially sensitive to stress. This is where the part of the brainstem called the medulla oblongata and the four cervical nerves that leave from it are located. The medulla oblongata directly regulates autonomic activity. Not only does it play a central role in maintaining life—controlling respiration, circulation, and digestion—but it's an important pathway of movement and sensation.

Autonomic balance is impaired if the medulla oblongata and other brain areas associated with the autonomic nervous system become tense. The hyperactivity of the sympathetic nervous system that is present during prolonged stress continues. And the tension in the medulla oblongata and sympathetic nervous system inhibits respiratory and circulatory function, so hot blood and energy rush toward the head. If ignored, this unrelieved tension can eventually lead to headache, insomnia, high blood pressure, and other problems.

The pivoting of your head on your neck during Brain Wave Vibration releases the heat and tension from this sensitive area, freeing your nervous system to resume its natural function. When your head is full of heat, it's also important to exhale that heat by continuously breathing out through your mouth. If you do this for even a minute, a great deal of heat will be expelled and you'll be able to feel the tension in your head and the back of your neck decrease.

According to a paper published in *Neuroscience Letters* in 2010, a joint study by the Korea Institute of Brain Science (KIBS) and Seoul National University (SNU) Hospital found a 56 percent reduction in stress and a 29 percent increase in blood dopamine levels among a group of Brain Wave Vibration practitioners versus a control group.

In another study, this one in Volume 2012 of *Evidence-Based Complementary and Alternative Medicine,* researchers from the University of London and the Korea Institute of Brain Science assessed the comparative effects of Brain Wave Vibration, Iyengar Yoga, and mindfulness training on mood, well-being, and immune function. The research team noted evidence of an "improvement in sleep [that] has been a common anecdotal report by Brain Wave Vibration practitioners, as has increase in energy and vitality."

Sleep affects the function of the autonomic nervous system, while at the same time, many of the physiological phenomena that occur during sleep, as well as our daily biorhythm, are regulated by this system. An improvement in sleep indicates better balance between the body's sympathetic and parasympathetic modes.

3 *Brain Wave Vibration changes brain matter.*

A study comparing a control group with people who'd done Brain Wave Vibration meditation for at least three years showed increased cortical thickness in the frontal and temporal lobes—centers of thinking, judgment, and emotional regulation—of the Brain Wave Vibration practitioners. This seems to indicate that Brain Wave Vibration may be effective for preventing dementia and other degenerative brain diseases, and may have an anti-aging effect. It could also be described as having a positive effect on brain development, including attention, memory, and emotional regulation. The results of the study were published in 2012 in the neuroscience journal *Social Cognitive and Affective Neuroscience.*

4 *Brain Wave Vibration strengthens the body's energy center.*

Tapping the lower abdomen is effective for strengthening the energy in that part of the body. Even in terms of physical structure, the lower abdomen is at the center of the body. The view of Eastern medicine is that vital energy collected in the lower abdomen—the Dahnjon, or energy center—circulates out to the entire body. Within the Dahnjon energy system, located two inches below the navel, is the meridian point called the *Kihae*, or "ocean of energy." This is precisely the place we focus on tapping when we do Brain Wave Vibration.

When you rhythmically tap your lower abdomen, alternating loosely held fists, it helps if you imagine that you're stirring up waves in an ocean of energy. Imagine those waves spreading to and warming your lower abdomen, then your whole body. If you do Brain Wave Vibration after you've increased your body temperature and blood/energy circulation by doing Plate Balancing and Toe Tapping, you'll experience more heat being generated in your lower abdomen. Your lower and upper back will be warmed and your body temperature will go up so much that you'll sweat.

Besides strengthening your energy center, tapping your lower abdomen aids digestion by stimulating the intestinal wall, relaxing and raising the temperature of the intestines. And the tapping vibration helps with detoxification by getting rid of food residue stuck in the bumps and curves of the intestines.

It's important, initially, to concentrate on tapping only the lower abdomen rather than randomly tapping here or there. Once your lower abdomen is sufficiently warm, it's all right to tap other places where you feel blockages, such as your lower back, chest, arms, and legs. After doing full-body tapping this way, you'll feel your whole body being refreshed. Not only does this open all the energy points, allowing energy to flow smoothly, but it also releases tension in knotted muscles and opens the pores to help your body secrete sweat and waste materials.

5 *Brain Wave Vibration restores the natural rhythm of life.*

When you do Brain Wave Vibration for a while, the hands tapping your lower abdomen end up rotating vertically while you move your head left and right horizontally. If you try to do this intentionally, your brain may feel slightly confused. The best approach is to focus on the sensations you feel in your body, not on your thoughts.

You'll feel some natural rhythm as you continue the simple movements of Brain Wave Vibration. If the movements feel awkward or in conflict with each other, stop shaking your head and focus on tapping your lower abdomen. When that becomes rhythmic and natural, start shaking your head again. Gently tapping your lower abdomen is the most basic movement for adjusting your body's energy balance. It's something you can do whenever you feel in need of stability and balance, whether you're exercising, working, or thinking. You'll feel great power in these simple movements.

If we focus on the simple and repeated beat of a drum or other percussion instrument, we're likely to find ourselves moving our feet and bobbing our heads to the beat without even being conscious of it. Later our shoulders and our upper body—our whole body—move to the beat. This happens when the natural rhythm within us awakens and finds expression. In just the same way, if you enter into the feeling of being yourself as you do Brain Wave Vibration, the rhythm of life within you will awaken and begin to express itself. Then you'll get a taste of joy and freedom much like what you experience when you dance intensely, entrusting your body to a powerful beat. And after you finish Brain Wave Vibration, you'll feel incredible stillness, peace, and joy of life welling up from within.

BRAIN WAVE VIBRATION
Q&A

Q *I get dizzy when I shake my head from side to side. What should I do?*

A When trying any unfamiliar exercise for the first time, it's natural to experience some slight discomfort as your body adapts. You might feel a little dizziness as you shake your head when you first learn Brain Wave Vibration. Stop moving and control your breathing as you rest with your chin tucked in slightly, and the dizziness will subside. Be careful not to shake your head too quickly or for too long at first. It will also help if you open your mouth slightly and continue to exhale the stagnant energy and air from your head and chest.

It's especially easy to feel dizzy if excessive work or stress has created severe tension in the cervical vertebrae or the back of your head, or if your chest feels constricted or you have a lot of blood in your head. If you have headaches, anemia, high blood pressure, or low blood pressure, be even more cautious and adjust the speed and duration of the movements appropriately. Even slow, gentle, back-and-forth movement is effective for releasing tension in the brain and cervical vertebrae; the motion doesn't have to be fast. Once you've gotten somewhat comfortable with the movement, try to increase the speed of the shaking a little bit—but don't overdo it.

Q
Do I need specific music for Brain Wave Vibration?

A
Strictly speaking, Brain Wave Vibration practice does not require music. It is about your own internal rhythms, not about moving to a beat as you would when you dance. However, music can be helpful when you begin. Obviously, very slow and sentimental music is not suitable for the vibration. The most effective music for Brain Wave Vibration is music with a strong basic beat, such as that found in many forms of traditional drumming. I find Korean samulnori to be especially effective because it awakens the brain with a lively combination of sounds from gongs and drums, generating a powerful vibration that you can feel throughout your body.

In addition to samulnori, percussive folk instruments from Africa and South America offer a simple, primitive repetition of sound that replicates the basic rhythms of life. Music is helpful to induce the proper state of mind for Brain Wave Vibration in the beginning, but as time goes by, the rhythm of the body should overpower the rhythm of the music. Be sure to focus inward at all times and allow your own rhythm to come forward.

LINKING THE 10-10-10 EXERCISE

You can do the three movements of the Solar Body Exercises in a sequence in 30 minutes. Investing just 30 minutes a day promotes a steady flow of energy and blood circulation throughout the body and strengthens the core, helping maintain a Solar Body state that's charged with natural healing power.

Some people worry about which exercise they should do first. Basically, there's no problem with doing the exercises in whatever order you feel is best for your physical condition and how you feel at the time. However, you can experience a greater effect if you adjust the sequence according to the time of day.

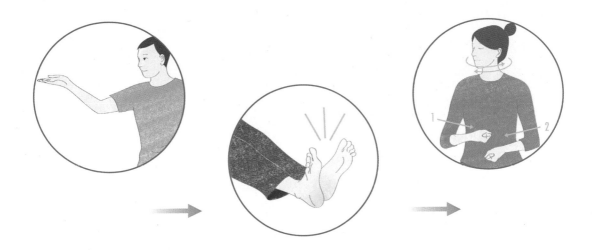

DURING THE DAY:
PLATE BALANCING > TOE TAPPING > BRAIN WAVE VIBRATION

This is the most common order for the 10-10-10 Exercise. We start with Plate Balancing to promote full-body energy and blood circulation, since we generally do a lot of activities in a standing posture during the day. Next, lying down comfortably to do Toe Tapping causes the energy and blood massing toward the head to sink into the lower body. And finally Brain Wave Vibration, done sitting down, purifies the brain and strengthens the power of the core in the lower abdomen, charging us with energy for the rest of the day.

IN THE MORNING:
TOE TAPPING > BRAIN WAVE
VIBRATION > PLATE BALANCING

Morning is when skeletal and muscular flexibility have declined, blood pressure increases, and body temperature drops. Rather than starting with Plate Balancing, which involves big movements in a standing posture, it's better to warm up the body with Toe Tapping and Brain Wave Vibration to develop the strength of the lower abdomen and legs. Especially for those who are physically weak, this sequence helps develop strength without being at all extreme.

It's easy to remember the morning sequence if you think about how you get out of bed. Just as you first sit up from your lying posture and then stand, start with Toe Tapping in a lying posture, then sit up and do Brain Wave Vibration. Finish by standing up for Plate Balancing.

You awaken the organs and cells of your body, develop your leg strength, and raise the temperature of your lower body as you do Toe Tapping. Next you awaken your brain and augment the power and heat in your lower abdomen with Brain Wave Vibration. When you stand to do Plate Balancing, your whole body is charged with energy and vitality, and you can feel your movements becoming more flexible and powerful. Applying the Solar Body Exercises in this sequence provides vitality for the day's activities by activating the sympathetic nervous system, which was relaxed during sleep.

IN THE EVENING:
PLATE BALANCING > BRAIN WAVE
VIBRATION > TOE TAPPING

In the evening, you need to slow your brain waves and relax your sympathetic nervous system to get ready for sleep. Imagine yourself being active and then going to bed, the opposite of what you do in the morning. Start by doing Plate Balancing in a standing position, sit to do Brain Wave Vibration, and finish by lying down for Toe Tapping.

You do the Plate Balancing first to release the tension your body has accumulated throughout the day, since this is when your body is hottest and most flexible. Relax the tension in your shoulders, chest, sides, and lower back by rotating your arms and waist. Then sit down and rock your brain from side to side, shaking off the day's stress and difficulties. As you tap your lower abdomen, pull down into your belly the hot energy that has risen during the day.

Finally, lie down in a comfortable position to do Toe Tapping, discharging through your mouth and toes all the weariness and stress energy built up during the day, purifying your energy. If you do the exercises in this order, your body and mind will easily relax and your brain waves will slow, allowing you to enjoy deep, restful sleep.

CREATE YOUR OWN EXERCISE ROUTINE

Linking the three exercises and doing them together for 30 minutes is the most effective, but you can also do them separately when you don't have the time to do them all at once.

It helps to strengthen your vitality during the day by doing Plate Balancing and Brain Wave Vibration, and to get a good night's sleep by doing Toe Tapping when you're getting ready for bed in the evening. It's also good to wake up your body in the morning by doing Toe Tapping in bed when you first awaken and open your eyes, or to recharge your power periodically with Plate Balancing and Brain Wave Vibration during the day.

And it's fine to do an exercise for as long as you want, depending on your physical condition. There's no limit that says you can do it for only 10 minutes. Even if you do Toe Tapping in the morning, you can also do it later as you sit watching TV, and you can repeat it to get ready for bed in the evening. Practice Plate Balancing or Brain Wave Vibration whenever you have extra time at home, at work, or during outdoor activities.

Observe the state of your body. Don't hesitate to stop what you're doing or thinking when you feel your vitality drop, or when stress makes your shoulders stiff or your head hot. You don't need to set aside a big chunk of time or put on your outdoor gear. You have the Solar Body Exercises. As you recharge, you'll be able to feel your body and mind overflowing with bright and powerful life energy.

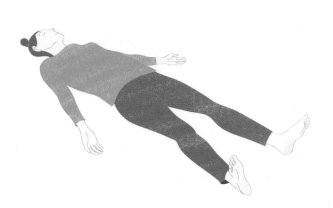
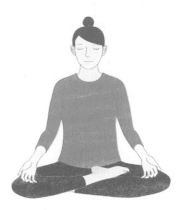

FEELING YOUR BODY HEAT

There's something important you should always do after the 10-10-10 Exercise, and that's to feel your body heat.

Close your eyes while lying down or in your seated position and try to feel your body heat. How has your body temperature changed? Try to feel what part of your body has gotten warmer and what part is cooler.

Being able to feel your body heat means that your consciousness is focused inside your body, so this is a great way to pull your consciousness inward after it's been directed outward for most of the day. What's more, feeling your body heat is an easy way to check the condition of your body and mind.

First check the state of your energy and blood circulation as you feel your body heat. You'll feel that your hands and feet are warmer and that your body temperature has risen after doing the 10-10-10 Exercise. This means your circulation has increased enough to supply energy and blood to all your extremities. Once your energy and blood circulation are invigorated, you'll feel tingling sensations here and there, as if all the cells have been activated.

Your lower abdomen and lower body will also feel warmer, your chest more comfortable, and your head lighter and more refreshed. You'll feel warm, powerful energy gradually condensing in the energy center in your lower abdomen. This means that you've developed Water-up, Fire-down circulation, the body's ideal energy state. It means that your body has recovered a natural balance of energy and blood circulation.

Now check your breathing as you feel your body heat. With the tension in your chest, back, shoulders, and abdomen relaxed after the 10-10-10 Exercise, you'll be able to feel your breath entering and leaving your body naturally and easily. Fresh air fills your lungs thanks to your more comfortable chest, and deep abdominal breathing happens automatically, thanks to your relaxed, warmer belly. The more deeply you breathe with your lower abdomen at this time, the more you'll feel powerful energy coming together as your lower abdomen grows warmer.

Those who've mastered this exercise actually feel as if air is entering their body all the way to their lower abdomen and leaving through the soles of their feet. In the Eastern practice of Tao, this is spoken of as the highest form of breathing, "sole breathing." Air isn't actually coming into the soles of the feet, but energy entering through the major meridian point in the middle of the sole makes it feel that way.

Finally, check the state of your mind as you feel your body heat. When you're suffering from stress during the day, you develop a feeling of constriction in your chest. Heat rises toward your head and chest. After doing the 10-10-10 Exercise, this heat sinks. It feels as if your stress has flown away and your once-constricted chest is now wide open.

Vitality returns to your body and mind when you blow away the stress—the depressing, stagnant energy weighing heavily on your chest—through Plate Balancing, with its big, circular arm movements. Your brain feels clearer and more tranquil when you brush off all negative thoughts through the shaking of Brain Wave Vibration. When you're lying down after having stagnant energy released through Toe Tapping, it feels as if all the cells in your body are living and breathing. Your body and mind are so light that you feel as if you're floating on a cloud, and you think, *This is the most comfortable, peaceful feeling in the world!*

When your chest feels tight and full of stress, when your mind is heavy and depressed, when dark, negative energy dominates you, try doing the 10-10-10 Exercise. Afterward, with your eyes closed and your consciousness focused in your lower abdomen, feel your body heat. You'll sense that your energy and blood circulation, breathing, and mind are all in an optimal state for maximizing your natural healing power. Your body will feel lighter, your mind refreshed.

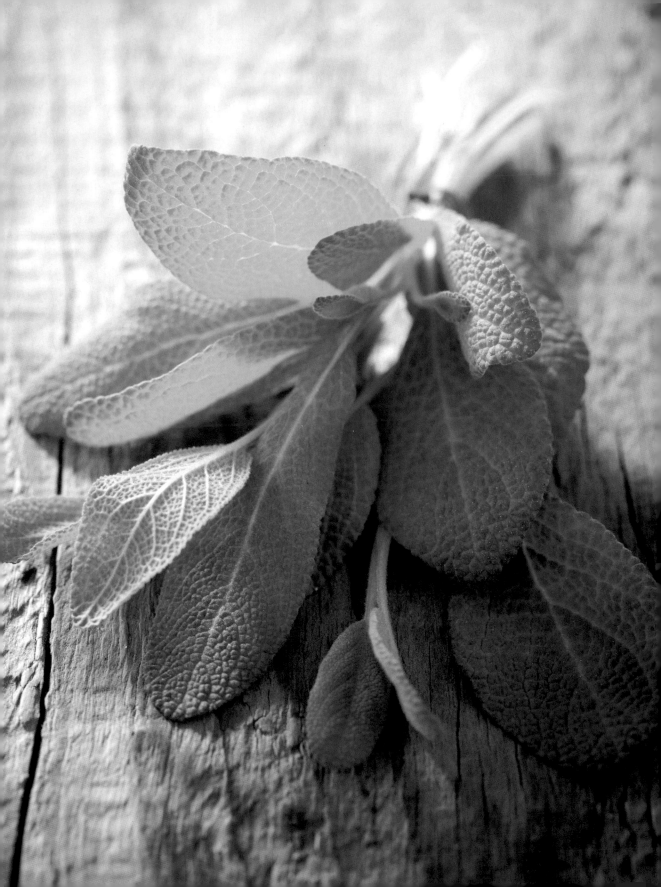

USING SOLAR HERBS

INTRODUCING SAGE

One day I broke off and slowly chewed a gray-green leaf from a sage plant I'd been given by a friend. At first the leaf tasted so bitter that I wanted to spit it out. The more I chewed it, though, the more the taste and the aroma seemed to cool my head and calm my mind. That's when I came to believe that this is a powerful, natural tool for creating a Solar Body—a marvelous brain refresher.

I've long been interested in herbs used for natural healing, so I'm in the habit of tasting plants that are said to be good for the body. Of these, sage is truly unique. Its powerful taste and aroma really wake up the brain. Do you remember the refreshing feeling in your mouth or the sense of your sinuses really opening up when you've chewed mint gum or sucked on a piece of herbal-flavored candy? The feeling you get when you chew sage leaf is dozens of times more powerful than that.

Slowly chew a sage leaf and you'll feel all the orifices in your face—your mouth, nose, eyes, even your ears—opening up. Every breath you take will send sage-scented air into your nasal cavity and your brain, making them feel incredibly refreshed. What's more, the more you chew the sage, the more you'll feel saliva filling your mouth. Viewed from the standpoint of energy training, saliva fills the mouth when your body has good energy and blood circulation. As you swallow the saliva, your abdomen and then your whole body will grow warmer. Sage is truly a miraculous healing herb that creates Water-up, Fire-down circulation, making the head cool and the abdomen warm.

I found that sage has countless beneficial properties. Its botanical name is *Salvia*, meaning "healthy" or "safe, whole." Native to the Mediterranean, sage has been known for its healing properties for thousands of years. In fact, sage supposedly was considered divine in ancient Greece and Rome. In modern times, it was named "Herb of the Year" in 2001 by the International Herb Association.

Its healing properties are so varied that it would be difficult to list them all. Sage has anti-inflammatory, disinfectant properties and has been widely used to treat inflammation of the mouth, gums, throat, and nasal passages, as well as to treat colds, fever, headache, cough, and asthma. It has been used for digestive symptoms, menstrual pain, and menopausal symptoms because it warms the abdomen. Sage also makes the head cool, and it has been used for brain-related symptoms such as memory loss, Alzheimer's disease, and difficulty concentrating. Besides adding flavor to food, sage has antimicrobial and preservative effects, aids in digestion, and masks unpleasant odors.

There's a reason I recommend sage for use with the Solar Body Method. Besides its ability to rapidly create a Water-up, Fire-down energy state, sage is extremely effective for waking the spirit and controlling the mind. Sage is unique in that it rouses the brain, uplifting and improving mood, and at the same time calms and settles the mind. In other words, it is effective for developing a Solar Body and creating a peaceful, bright mind.

Slowly chewing sage greatly helps us watch and control our thoughts, emotions, and cravings. Our brains have a tendency to thirst for what's novel and stimulating. That's why we buy new cars and clothes, why we want to journey to places with ever more wonderful sights, and why we're so impressed with a delicious food tasted for the first time. In serious cases, the brain's needs result in an addiction to alcohol, drugs, games, or other things.

It's ultimately the action of the brain that either causes or controls such needs. The key, then, is to discover how to lead the brain, enabling it to get a good handle on its desires. Ceaselessly craving stimulus, your brain will begin to listen to you if you offer other things to satisfy it. I felt hope for this as I developed a training method using sage. The flavor and aroma of this plant are powerful enough to shock the brain. It makes you wonder whether any other plant has such power.

Let's say someone wants to quit smoking. He's tried several times, but he's always ended up kneeling in submission before his cravings. So his confidence keeps dropping, and he tells himself that he's too weak-willed to keep the promises he made to himself. But if he slowly chews sage, as his brain is roused he'll realize that he needs to control his negative desires and habits. In other words, he wakes up and pays attention. And as the aroma refreshes his brain, his craving for tobacco abates considerably. His mind is calmed by the sage, which has provided stimulation more powerful than his cravings.

Sage can help us develop concentration as well. When your brain feels heavy and constricted and your concentration drops, when you feel depressed and long to feel refreshed, slowly chew a sage leaf. The crispness of your breath will make you feel better as your brain is refreshed.

Native Americans practiced smudging by burning the leaves and branches of sagebrush, a sage of the genus *Artemisia*, to purify negative energy. "Negative energy" could be some harmful desire or information in your brain. When you breathe in the unique aromas that comes from burning any type of sage, your brain is refreshed and you develop the willpower to calm and control the negativity.

A founding myth of Korea, where I was born, tells of Ungnyeo (Bear Woman), the mother of Dahngun, the founder of the Korean nation. She ate only mugwort and garlic while she stayed in a cave, training to awaken to her original nature. Also of the genus *Artemisia*, mugwort has properties quite similar to those of sage, so in Eastern medicine it is used for moxibustion thermotherapy, and also as an oral medication. People commonly use mugwort both as an herbal therapy and as a food.

Could Ungnyeo have chosen to eat mugwort because, like sage, it helps control emotions and cravings and awakens the brain? I confidently recommend sage as the best herb for transforming body and mind, and developing a Solar Body. It is excellent not only for recovering natural healing power, but also for developing willpower and concentration and for reviving a bright spirit.

HOW TO USE THE SOLAR HERB

Sage is an amazing herbal medicine, affordable for anyone because it can be raised at home or purchased at an ordinary grocery store. It can be used as a seasoning for cooking or boiled as a tea, and the dried leaves can be burned for use in smudging to purify energy. But I think the best way to experience its powerful effects is to consume it directly by chewing raw leaves. About one leaf a day is an appropriate amount to use for the sage training method described below.

1. Place a fresh sage leaf in your mouth, then very slowly and gently chew it with your front teeth at the tip of your tongue. A bitter taste will begin to spread in your mouth. Chew with your front teeth for about three minutes, then slowly chew with your back teeth. When saliva fills your mouth, swallow it. You can continue this for about 10 minutes, or up to an hour.

2. Try to feel the changes in your body as you slowly chew the sage. As your nose, eyes, and ears open up, your breathing will become fresher and deeper, and your lower abdomen—your whole body—will grow warmer.

3. Feel the changes in your mind, too. You'll sense your brain being refreshed, your heart growing brighter and calmer. Visualize your energy gradually growing brighter, shining like the sun, as you offer yourself positive, hopeful affirmations that will give you strength.

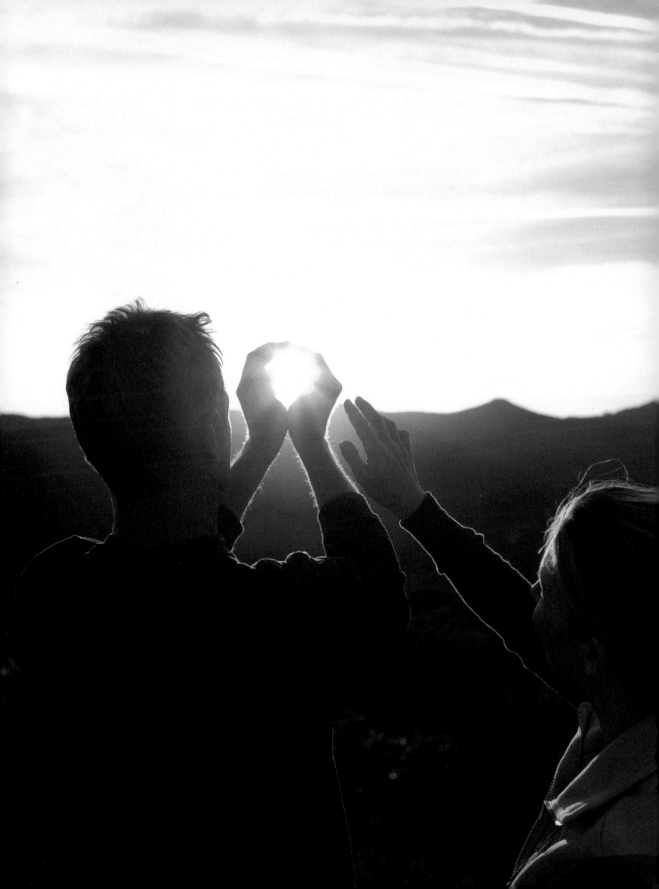

CHAPTER 3

LIVING AS A SOLAR BODY

FIND YOUR OWN
RHYTHM OF LIFE

RECOVER YOUR INNER SENSE

So far I've talked about body temperature, breathing, and the observation of the mind as three keys for recovering natural healing power. I've introduced the three components of the Solar Body Method—Sunlight Meditation, Solar Energy Circuit Training, and Solar Body Exercises—as techniques anyone can use. But even powerful, effective principles and exercises are useless unless you experience them yourself. More than anything else, I hope you will experience the Solar Body Method personally.

Start with a week, then try to keep following the Solar Body Method for a month, and then three months. If you continue steadily for about three months, this will become a wonderful routine for starting or ending your day—and in that process you'll experience amazing changes in your body and mind.

When you're mentally overloaded or feeling under the weather, stop what you're doing and try Solar Energy Circuit Training. Try to feel the circuits acting on your body, positively changing your energy in surprisingly rapid and powerful ways, and recharging you with vitality. And try to do Solar Body Exercises whenever you get the chance. It's good if you can do all three, but it's also fine to do any one of them for as little as five minutes. After doing the exercise that's right for your situation, try to feel your body heat as you breathe naturally, deeply, and slowly.

By repeating the simple exercises and meditations of the Solar Body Method, you can create healthy vital changes within yourself. When your thoughts and emotions settle down and complete silence finds you, you'll suddenly realize how beautiful a being you are. The realization will come that you are a precious, complete being—neither better nor worse than others, but incomparable.

It's the realization that you're precious and valuable *as you are*, not because you've successfully completed a major project, earned a lot of money, or been loved. It's the realization that you're a precious, valuable being even if you've failed at business, ruined an important project, or have yet to be successful after years of attempting to quit smoking or lose weight. The realization will come to you that you will always gain strength and begin again by trusting in the great life force within you—in the goodness of nature, which cares for all things with infinite love—and by connecting with the infinite source of life.

This is a time when you have found your own life rhythm. The life within you has bloomed fully with its inherent rhythm, and you feel complete oneness with yourself. This is when an environment has been created that allows your natural healing power to act most vigorously. This is when your body recovers health as it finds its original balance, when happiness fills your heart and your soul experiences deep peace.

Feeling life's rhythm in our bodies and restoring natural healing power isn't something we need to learn. This is something we've received from nature, not something that was artificially created. The problem is that our educational and social systems have made us grow more distant from this sense of life. Having been trained to find our value in external recognition or assessments—to depend on externalities even for the most essential issues of life, like health and happiness—we've lost the sense of life that exists inside us.

As the gift of the Creator, natural healing power is ours. That's why no special method is needed for recovering it. There are no perfect methods, no matter how effective or powerful they may be. What is perfect is our sense of life itself.

The Solar Body Method isn't perfect; it's only another method, a primer or trigger. In time, when you've recovered your sense of connecting with the great life force within you and have rediscovered your natural healing power through this method, you'll be able to create a variety of exercises that are right for you. What I hope is that you'll realize through experience that the perfect sense of life is already within you—that a great healer exists in you. It's not a question of knowledge, but of experience.

In the course of awakening your senses and recovering your natural healing power, you will develop the attention to carefully watch all the phenomena arising inside you—your thoughts, emotions, and ideas—as well as your body. And through that process you will develop the ability to identify where and how your body is uncomfortable, what emotions easily entrap you and when, and what aspect of your consciousness is not yet free.

This is the beginning of change. Healing and change start with being aware of what needs to be healed and to change. Change begins when you become aware of the discomfort and lack of freedom in your body, of emotions that you hadn't been aware of before. It begins as small changes, but repetition soon leads to the recovery of health and the correction of habits. Continuous self-development follows, and positive change spreads like a wave into the whole of your life.

DISCOVER YOUR INNER SUN

Rarely will you find a place where you can feel nature, and the sun, as much as you can in Sedona, Arizona, where I live. When you climb a hill covered with juniper trees at sunrise and see the morning light shining over the desert, you feel with your whole body that the sun is the source of life. The land, grass, and plants awaken vividly with the golden morning sunshine to start the day.

Today a new sun drives away last night's darkness. This is a powerful symbol of hope and regeneration. I begin the day with this reverent awareness of the universe, which has continued without missing a day since the sun and the earth were born, and I'm grateful for the absolute love and power of nature, which has permitted me this new day.

Watch the sunrise and the sunset often, if you can. Walk in the warm sunshine, and take the time to do Sunlight Meditation frequently. Spend lots of time with the sun in this way and you'll be deeply moved by nature, which cares for all things in the universe through an absolute love, free of all prejudice. The natural healing power of your body will grow stronger as you're moved by the power of nature, which grants order and harmony to all things. And the mind inside you will shine all the brighter.

A Solar Body resembles the sun. He creates his own health and his own light. He knows that he holds the source of infinite energy within himself and is always ready to return to that source for strength. And he always illuminates his surroundings and the world with positive energy, as the sun illuminates all things.

A Solar Body is also someone who actively discovers the sun within herself—that is, a mind bright like the sun, and one who actively uses that mind. Everyone has that mind. Everyone can discover and use that mind. Just as the sun shines through when the clouds clear away, so, too, that mind is always shining very brightly when all the thoughts and emotions obscuring it clear away.

Once you've seen and felt that mind, don't hold back. Use that mind actively! Illuminate and heal your body with that sun-like mind. Shine its light into every nook and cranny of your life to create the change you have so desired. Shining the light of that mind on those around you and on the world, make this world a better place.

You will be able to live as your authentic self when you find that infinite source of energy and that mind, bright and shining like the sun. Then you won't need to become anyone other than yourself. You won't need to depend on externals for your health and happiness, and you won't need to look outside yourself to find passion and hope for life.

A SOLAR BODY STORY

In Korea, there is someone known as "the woman who lives on water alone." Her name is Ae-ran Yang, and she is 65 this year. Her amazing story has been published in several books and introduced through Korean TV and newspapers. Fascinated by her mode of life, which is so different from those of ordinary people, I met with her twice and spoke with her at length.

One day in her thirteenth year, Yang says, she started to dislike eating food. She says she couldn't eat even though she tried. When she swallowed the porridge or fruit her shocked family forced her to eat, she would throw it all up. With the help of her older brother, who was studying medicine, she went all over visiting large hospitals and famous doctors, but they couldn't find a cause for her condition, and it didn't improve.

Since then, she has lived for 52 years on water alone. Although she does very occasionally drink juice made by gently blending watermelon in a mixer, even that is rare. Since she doesn't eat anything, she almost never defecates. Once every month or two, Yang says, she defecates in mouse-dropping-size quantities.

Biologically and medically, it is known that human beings must consume a certain amount of calories to survive. Running contrary to such common sense, Yang's story is probably hard to believe, but it is a fact that she lives without eating food. She hardly sleeps and barely drinks a liter of water a day—small sips, just enough to quench her thirst. She says that small quantities of water are enough for her to feel full, and that she has no desire for food.

Many people are shocked and worried by her emaciated frame. She appears to be little more than bones and weighs only about 44 pounds. But she says she feels very healthy. It doesn't seem like she'd have much energy, but her voice is strong and she passes right by ordinary folks when she goes for hikes. She doesn't often wear socks, even in cold weather, because her body is hotter than other people's bodies.

What she likes best is walking in nature. She walks an average of two to three hours a day. Yang says she walks all day long when she gets the chance, and that her body and mind are filled with vitality when she goes where there are trees and grass and birds and water. The energy others get from food, Yang seems to get from nature.

Ae-ran Yang is also called by the name "Loving Mother," for her insight and wisdom. I offer here a message she'd like to convey:

"Disease" does not exist in the seat of a person's Original Mind. When they get a great shock or are hurt, people don't wipe these things away quickly, but instead hold them in their hearts and keep making them worse. If they experience a similar situation or even see a similar person, they again pull out and obsess over those memories as if they were precious treasures held close to the chest. "Disease" refers to a shock or hurt developed in that way, one that comes to light because it can no longer be hidden. And everyone easily acknowledges it once a disease starts to show itself.

In the seat of the Origin, however, there is no sickness and no place that hurts.

Although Yang's story is so extreme as to be unbelievable, it shows the infinite potential of the Solar Body. It shows the possibility of more actively using the life energy contained in air, water, and the sun instead of depending completely on the energy that comes through food.

We have a fixed idea that higher organisms exist higher up in the food chain. Viewed from an energy perspective, however, the higher we rise in the food chain, the greater is our dependence on other organisms to maintain our own life. Conversely, the lower we go, the lower is that level of dependence. A plant lives on air, water, and sunlight alone. If we develop the ability to absorb and use energy itself, we will be able to maintain and manage our health much more effectively, without depending on the external environment and external conditions.

I'm not trying to say that we should only drink water and should eat no food, like Ae-ran Yang, or that we should photosynthesize, like plants. What I am trying to say is that, if we open ourselves to the life energy that exists infinitely in nature, and if we make active use of this personally, we'll be able to live much healthier lives than we do now. Globally, a sustainable new culture will be possible.

If we could obtain energy directly from solar energy—an infinite quantity of which exists in the universe—we would be able to maintain rich, healthy lives while using fewer resources and less energy than we do now, including food. We would create less waste, and the conflicts that occur around the possession and distribution of resources would decline.

Is this something that's possible only for beings like Superman, who rose above the atmosphere when his energy declined and recharged himself on sunlight? I don't think so. By awakening the sense for balance that exists within us, the lives of Solar Bodies can open a new way ahead, enabling the human race to evolve in a better direction and making possible a more harmonious civilization on this earth.

BECOME THE BEGINNING OF CHANGE

HOW DOES CHANGE BEGIN?

There's something I'd really like to ask of you as we come to the end of this book. If you've felt anything while reading this book, please put it into practice, even if it's a small thing. Please let change start with you.

Recovering the natural healing power and the goodness of human nature within us to create our own health, happiness, and peace doesn't end at an individual level. This is a wonderful seed for a new, peaceful, sustainable global culture.

Many of the activities we pursue, the resources we consume, and the waste products we create are the products of our desire to make our bodies a little more comfortable and carefree. Whether it's food, exercise, music, alcohol, sex, drugs—whatever the stimulus—ultimately what we seek is a feeling of satisfaction. In the end, though, true satisfaction arises from a balance of healthy, harmonious energy. And that harmonious, balanced energy is the core of the natural healing power I've talked about in this book.

That sense of satisfaction is unlikely to be sustained when it depends on external stimulation and isn't based on harmonious and balanced energy. That's why we end up searching for stronger stimuli, use more energy and resources, and create more waste. If we look at our mode of living and speak about it honestly, we have to acknowledge that our satisfaction means stress for the planet.

Recovering a sense of balanced energy and maintaining our health in a natural way doesn't only signify a reduction in the resources that go directly toward sustaining health and treating disease. It will bring overall change to lifestyles that currently revolve around stimuli and satisfaction, and as a result it will contribute to increasing the natural healing power of the earth itself.

Once our natural healing power is restored, our eyes will naturally be opened to see the interconnection of our individual decisions with the world as a whole. Just as waves cannot be separated from water, an inseparable whole is formed by us individuals and all humanity, and by humanity and the earth itself. The choices I make each moment, great and small, have an effect on the future of humanity and the earth.

Denying that all life is one and destroying the earth itself—the basis of our survival—is obviously seen as foolish by those whose natural healing power has been restored. Just as you voluntarily avoid foods and habits that damage your health once your body's senses have been restored, so you no longer do things that harm the health and harmony of the planet.

The deeper your own connection to yourself grows, the more you grow to have a deep interest in and affection for all life, and an attitude of passion and dedication. And very naturally you sense that the problems of humanity are your own problems. When you have a Solar Body that creates its own health and happiness, you cannot avoid the realization that *you* are the one to save the earth and humanity. And so you come to live the life of a Solar Body, helping others to achieve the same realization.

SOLAR BODY FOR THE PLANET

The changes that appear in each of our lives as we recover our human nature may not, in fact, be that big. It's not like we all have to become saints in a single day, or gain miraculous healing abilities. This might manifest itself in a kindly smile for the person sitting next to you on the subway. It could appear in teaching Plate Balancing to a colleague who has been complaining of shoulder pain because of many hours spent working at a computer. Regardless of whether our countries are the same or different, our faith or attitudes toward religion the same or different, our lifestyles or tendencies the same or different, this is about becoming a little more friendly with one another. It's about not chasing after the body's needs and tastes but controlling them to avoid overeating, and it's about making choices that contribute to the whole even if we suffer some loss when our interests conflict with those of the whole. It is, literally, about becoming a good person.

Such changes are truly internal, and therefore they don't require us to wait until politics, economics, institutions, infrastructure, or industrial structure change. They can happen right now if we wake up and pay attention, and choose. They're changes that are fundamental and yet very gentle, quiet, and inexpensive.

These changes are the key to solving everything from individual problems around the world—like obesity and other lifestyle diseases—to the global environmental crisis and political/religious conflicts. They are, in fact, the key to creating a truly peaceful and sustainable world. The changes within each of us will alter the choices we make in our everyday lives, impacting everything in society and bringing meaningful, positive change.

Earlier in this book, I described 97.7 degrees F (36.5 degrees C) as the temperature of recovery and recharge and 99.5°F (37.5°C) as the temperature of vitality and passion. Our bodies and minds overflow with vitality when the temperature of our bodies and minds is that of passion. There's one more thing I want to stress for maintaining that state, and that thing is hope. If the three exercises of the Solar Body Method act as kindling for increasing body temperature, then hope could be said to be kindling for increasing the temperature of the mind. We become ambitious and develop confidence when we have hope. Solar Bodies are individuals who live passionate lives with the hope they've found in themselves. They are people who share hope and passion with those around them and enliven the world.

As long as I can find hope in myself, there is hope for the future of the earth and the human race. If I fail to discover hope in myself, there is no hope for the earth or the human race. If I discover the goodness of human nature in myself, I can find it in the entire human race. If I fail to discover it in myself, I can't expect it from anyone else, either.

I'd like to make a suggestion: whichever of the components of the Solar Body Method you practice, do it with boldness and great purpose. When you do Toe Tapping, think of it as the beginning of the restoration of natural healing power in your neighbors and in the earth, not just something you're doing for your own health. Think of the bright mind inside you growing greater with each breath you take as you feel your body heat after Brain Wave Vibration, and think of it helping you to make and follow through on better choices. Think of becoming a Solar Body as a way to save the planet.

Do these exercises for a month, for three months, for a year. The more steadily you repeat them, the more positive changes you will experience in your life, and the more you'll develop a passionate desire to take those changes deep into the center of your life—and to share them widely. Acting positively in response to that passion, let's make the world healthier, more peaceful, and more sustainable through the changes that start in ordinary people like you and me.

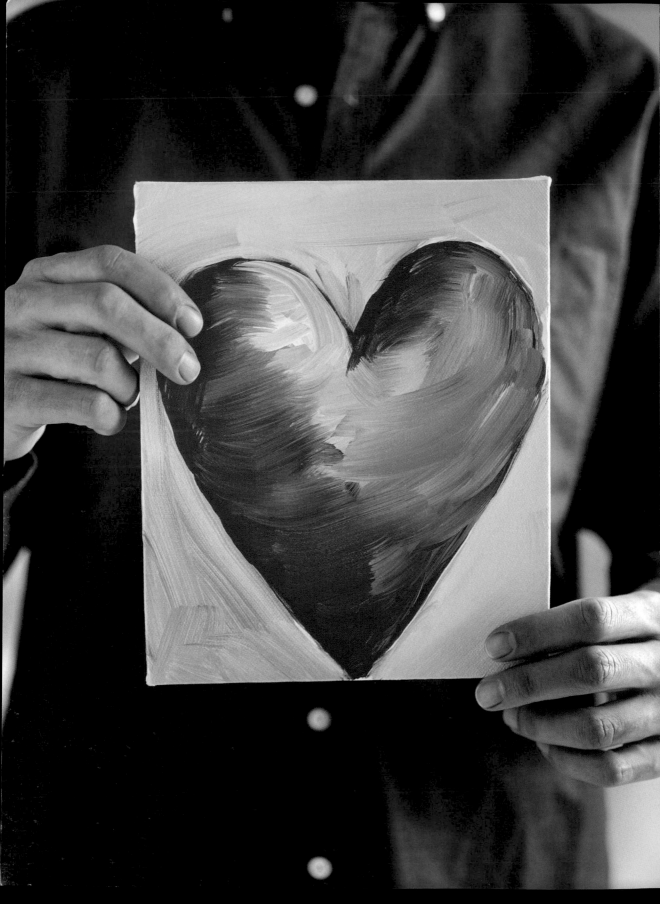

CHAPTER 4

STORIES OF HEALING AND EMPOWERMENT

SOLAR BODY METHOD ENERGIZED ME.

Beauty Swe
Internal Medicine Physician
Pasadena, California

As a result of the Solar Body Method, the feeling of energy, joy, and peace the whole day is so obvious to me. I've never felt this way before. I do it in the early morning and the energy lasts through bedtime.

Mentally and physically I have grown to be more loving and peaceful and have a more "flexible" brain and heart. The method gives you discipline and a purpose to your life and your days, and it gives you satisfaction and confidence and respect for yourself—that you are doing something good every day for your body and mind.

I have had a very bad cervical spine problem, and my orthopedic doctor recommended surgery. I had a ligament tear. With this simple exercise, I have been able to go back to my jogging, full of energy every day, even with my busy 16-hour workday. I was also impressed at how my heart rate, blood pressure, and respiratory rate went down over a three-week period.

I recommend these exercises to my patients, and I've found that older people with joint pain and arthritis improve their flexibility and are able to go back to their gardening. People with back pain and work injuries are walking straighter without the use of pain medication, and some no longer need surgery. People who are depressed or angry become more cheerful and smile more.

A friend who had a stroke stayed at my house to recover after being discharged from the hospital because there was no one to take care of her. She was assigned physical therapy, and I also showed her the 10-10-10 Exercise. She could do one rep of Plate Balancing the first day and then increased, one by one. After 10 days she could do nine repetitions. Her mobility improved and she had a positive attitude, whereas many stroke survivors tend to feel depressed. She got so much better that after two weeks she stopped her physical therapy sessions and focused on the Solar Body Method. She also went home, because she felt able to take care of herself.

PLATE BALANCING ALLEVIATED MY ARTHRITIS SYMPTOMS.

Hye-yeong Shin
Seoul, South Korea

After opening a home outfitters specialty store in 2009, I was so busy with work that I barely left the counter for two and a half years. In 2012, I was even introduced in one national economic weekly as a successful small business owner. However, I had to pay with my body the price for having worked so hard.

On my feet all day, I found that more and more of my body was hurting—my shoulders, my ankles, and my lower back. My joints ached so much that there wasn't a pain-free place in my body. When I went to the hospital, they told me I had rheumatoid arthritis, and that my joints would grow stiffer unless I started taking medication. I did bring home medication, but I suffered from reflux esophagitis, so I couldn't take it. The inflammation became very severe as a result, so my anxiety as well as my physical pain increased. Even taking someone's hand hurt.

On top of that, two years ago I developed degenerative arthritis in my neck, lower back, and ankles, so I couldn't walk properly. The doctor said the arthritis in my ankles was so severe that unless I had surgery right away, they would eventually have to amputate my leg. I was so shocked that when my husband called after the consultation, I couldn't talk about it honestly with him. He kept asking what was wrong. Crying, I finally told him. But there was no guarantee I'd be able to walk even if I had surgery, so he said, "Just come home. Let's find another way." Together we began searching for methods of natural healing.

I started yoga, breathing practices, and meditation, which is when I learned about Plate Balancing. I did this exercise and found that my joints felt more relaxed, and my whole body seemed refreshed. I had the intuition, *Oh, this will be really good for my joint health*. I've done Plate Balancing daily since then. Health clubs, swimming, and other exercises cost a lot of money. I'm busy running my store, so Plate Balancing has been good because I can easily take a moment to do it anytime and anywhere. It has been a perfect for me because I can rotate my joints, including my wrists, shoulders, lower back, and hips. I've practiced 10 minutes a day for the last two years—at home, at the store, and even while on a walk.

About three months after I started, I felt that my body was improving. When a year had passed, I felt completely better. I could run as well as walk. Previously, I couldn't bend forward because of my lower back disc problem, and I had trouble rotating my neck because of neck disc problems. Now I can freely rotate my neck and lower back. My shoulder pain has vanished, and symptoms of arthritis in my wrists and ankles have disappeared. My flexibility has improved so much that I can sit on the floor with my legs spread 180 degrees. I've lost 20 pounds, too.

My husband said, "You couldn't even walk properly or lift a spoon because of your painful fingers. It's truly miraculous that you're so healthy now."

Although it looks simple, Plate Balancing is a smart exercise that uses all the body's joints and their surrounding muscles. Since I've recovered health and vitality through Plate Balancing, I've been recommending the exercise to my family, and even to customers I meet at our store.

MY BODY BECAME ALIGNED AGAIN.

Peter Marsh
Yoga Instructor
Los Angeles, California

Before I started doing the Solar Body Method, I had hip pain and needed a walking stick due to an accident. I could walk on flat surfaces, but stairs were really painful. My doctor prescribed muscle relaxers and pain medication; it was that bad. The pain completely disappeared after three days of training, and I was able to walk without assistance and even run up stairs.

After 30 days of daily training, I started experiencing body alignment correction. My left leg had always been stiff, shorter than my right leg, and my left little toe couldn't touch the floor when I did Toe Tapping. After about 30 days, I started getting a heavy feeling around my left knee that released, and my left toe started to touch the floor. I also have more mental clarity and focus now, and emotionally I feel more at peace.

While doing Plate Balancing, an image flashed into my mind. When my hand rotated over my head, it looked as if the energy in the upper part of my brain was getting brighter, and when my hand swept down at waist level, the lower part of my brain was getting brighter. At another time, a different image came to me. When my hand swept overhead, my seventh chakra was awakening; and when I reached downward, the energy of my feet, legs, and first chakra awakened. Spiraling through the entire movement, all seven chakras were becoming harmonized.

SOLAR BODY METHOD IS MY BEST STRESS RELIEVER.

Dana Hurlock
Denver, Colorado

Since I started practicing the Solar Body Method, I believe I have greater flexibility in my lower back and hips. I have also been sleeping a lot better. My headaches are down to maybe one a month, I think due to relaxing during Toe Tapping and Brain Wave Vibration. I also have increased mobility in my shoulders. I feel that mentally and emotionally, I am more stable. Doing the training in the morning will usually set a good pace for the day. I start out relaxed, energized, and focused and can face any situation with little difficulty. The stresses of everyday life are easier to deal with. When things seem to spiral out of control, it is easier to calm myself and realize what is causing turmoil and work to resolve it. Toe Tapping in the evening helps calm my mind for sleep.

SOLAR BODY METHOD RESTORED MY "CAN-DO" SPIRIT.

Jessica Fleischman
Babylon Village, New York

When I started the Solar Body Method, I wanted to feel more confident and be able to tackle my daily stressors. I wanted to be able to wake up in the morning and feel refreshed. During the three weeks of the training, I lost three pounds. I have more stamina, and my circulation has improved, even in cold weather. My overall strength and musculature have improved, especially my arm and trapezius muscles. I tend to be double-jointed in all of my joints, but the Plate Balancing exercise, by relieving any shoulder tightness and strengthening my muscles, is preventing dislocation and shoulder blade overlap and pain. As a nurse, this is something I can teach my clients as an alternative therapy for arthritic pain.

This method has also helped me deal with insomnia and anxious thoughts. Doing this allows me to concentrate, and I can get more work done after I do my exercises. I also felt elevation of mood, almost as if weight had been lifted off my shoulders. The Solar Body Method provided an outlet for me to refocus my energy during a very rough time in my life. I am starting to feel a more spiritual connection within myself. During the whole process, I have seen growth in my ability to focus inward and reshape my mentality of "I can't. I won't" to "I can, and I will." Truly inspiring!

THIS EXERCISE IS LIKE MAGIC!

Debbie Borgia
Babylon Village, New York

After practicing the Solar Body Method for three weeks, I lost six pounds. When I do it, I reconnect with my body. I could feel the tension in my neck and shoulders when I quieted my mind. When my mind was quiet, I almost naturally relaxed and let go of my worries. Afterward I felt calm. Also, my energy level improved. I realized, *Don't allow yourself to stay in a place where you feel low. Move—change your energy.* Plate Balancing makes me happy. Doing Plate Balancing with plates makes me feel like a child: happy, silly, with not a care in the world!

More than once I had a headache when I started doing the exercises. Afterward, my headache was slight or had disappeared—like magic! Unreal! Instead of reaching for Tylenol when I have a headache, I realized, *Train!* Don't play into your pain or discomfort. A small amount of exercise changes your mind and your body condition like magic!

I monitored my temperature pre- and post-exercises. I've noticed that after 30 minutes, my temperature increased 0.6 degree Fahrenheit, which interests me because my temperature before the training was always as low as 97°F. I never have a temp. I learned that my state of mind is directly linked with my body's condition. I need to train daily to keep a healthy balance. During

Plate Balancing, I reflected on infinity as I was doing the movement. I realized that my possibilities are infinite. If I want it, create it.

I FEEL EVEN MORE ENERGETIC THAN I DID 20 YEARS AGO.

Joel Pierre-Louis
New York, New York

I began the Solar Body Method in 2013, one month after my retirement as a psychiatrist. I retired to take care of my health. I had high blood pressure and low thyroid, and I was prediabetic. I did not realize how sick I was until I started the program. I was stiff, clumsy, weak, and quite tense. I was about 30 pounds overweight.

Through the Solar Body Method, my body became looser and stronger, and I lost about 23 pounds. Even with medication, my blood pressure hadn't been controlled, but now it's as low as a young person's. My blood pressure is like that of a baby, my physician said. My blood sugar is good, my thyroid condition improved.

Over a year, I have changed for the better. I am more physically fit; I feel even more energetic than I did 20 years ago. I am very surprised. I am doing things that I never dreamed I would be able to do. Most importantly, I have more control over my mind and body. I control my appetite, and I'm more disciplined in my daily life. I feel mentally stronger, able to focus, to concentrate better and control my thought process. Emotionally, I feel more optimistic—that life has a purpose for me. I'm no longer anxious and worried. I feel more at ease with my fellows. I'm enjoying life to its fullest.

I'm teaching this method to a few elderly people, including my sister, cousins, and friends. I encourage all my acquaintances to practice the Solar Body Method. This training is completely integrated into my life. I don't see my life without it. I will continue for the rest of my life.

TOE TAPPING HELPED IMPROVE MY EYESIGHT.

Jun-bong Jang
Seoul, South Korea

It was in the late summer of 2012 when I started doing Toe Tapping. Returning home from golfing one day, I was carrying my clubs into the house when I collapsed into a sitting position. I'd heard that at around age 70 one's knees and legs become weaker, and I discovered that this wasn't something that just happened to other people. It wasn't easy to go up and down the stairs in my two-story apartment, either.

About that time, Ilchi Lee, the author of this book, recommended that I try Toe Tapping. I immediately started doing 200 repetitions every day. It took about two minutes to do them, and at first even that felt boring. But figuring that I might as well keep at it, I continued doing Toe Tapping whenever I had the opportunity. After about two months, my leg and knee strength had improved considerably, and I felt more agile. I play tennis every Wednesday, and the following day my thighs and calves always used to feel tight; occasionally I'd get cramps. All such symptoms disappeared about three months after I started Toe Tapping. I was able to sleep well, too. And with more strength in my legs, I could drive the golf ball farther! I really have fun doing Toe Tapping now that I've felt these effects.

I gradually increased the number of repetitions to 500, and then to 1,000. I now regularly do 1,000 when I go to bed at night and 1,000 in bed before I get up in the morning. Occasionally I do Toe Tapping as I watch TV during the evening news or listen to music on the radio. This way I can easily do about 3,000 repetitions a day, even if I do them slowly. Now if I skip even a day, my body feels a bit stiff and uncomfortable, and I get the feeling that I've forgotten something important.

Although I began Toe Tapping because of my knees, I've become healthier in every way. My symptoms of cerebral infarction, diabetes, kidney disease, and cirrhosis of the liver improved. The right side of my head had hurt for a long time, so I did up to 5,000 repetitions a day and the pain disappeared after about three months. The heels of my feet had cracked and my toenails turned black because I had severe diabetes, and that cleared up while I continued doing Toe Tapping.

When you get older, the inside of your mouth is often dry. My mouth began to fill with saliva two to three months after I started Toe Tapping. They say this is because the energy and blood circulation in my body has improved. And I used to suffer from trouble with bowel movements, but that has been resolved, too. The greatest effect of Toe Tapping is improved eyesight. About a year and a half after I started, the letters on road signs looked clear to me even without glasses. I've been doing Toe Tapping close to nine years now, and these days I enjoy playing golf and tennis without wearing glasses.

People in their late 60s or early 70s naturally talk a lot about health. People I hadn't seen in a while would tell me that my face was much brighter and that I looked very healthy, and they'd ask whether something good had happened or if I was taking medication. When that happened, I'd introduce Toe Tapping and teach people the basics. They've all been deeply impressed with its effects.

One friend had to go to the bathroom every two hours, and he'd often wake in the middle of the night. These days, he gets about five hours of sound sleep. He says the exercise is effective for dealing with prostate problems. Another friend said that his head is clearer and his concentration better. One friend, senior to me, had trouble walking beginning at age 86, so he'd ride a cart for golfing; a caddy placed his ball on the tee. He also stammered when he spoke. As a result of doing foot baths and Toe Tapping at my recommendation every morning and evening for more than four years, at age 90 he now not only walks to play golf, but he speaks very well, too.

There's one thing I've realized as I've continued to do Toe Tapping. Although it's good to do this and that—exercise and spiritual practices—if I don't have time for everything, I can get a greater effect when I stick with one thing and do it with perseverance. Through Toe Tapping, my body is being renewed every day, and my movements are actually becoming more agile. I just hope that my experiences will help others, too.

I IMPROVED FLEXIBILITY AND RELIEVED JOINT PAIN.

Lyn Miller
Katy, Texas

As a result of the Solar Body Method, my hands have almost completely stopped having the tingling and numbness I had experienced for over 10 years. Even though I've had stiffness and swelling from rheumatoid arthritis, now my shoulders no longer "click" when I move them. My hips do not have pain. Even my back is more flexible. My posture has improved, and I have increased stamina and vitality. Any initial stiffness I have goes away as I do the training. My legs are stronger, more toned, and more flexible.

I am also calmer and more peaceful. I am able to remain calm in difficult situations. I have always remained calm on the outside, but now I am calm on the inside! If I feel fatigue as I begin my training for the day, I am always refreshed when I finish. My focus is greatly improved. I am more productive at work and more attentive to my family and also myself. Part of the benefit is from committing to regular practice. Making the decision to give this method priority in my life helped me to overcome a plateau I had reached in my yoga practice.

ACKNOWLEDGMENTS

I would like to extend my sincere gratitude to all who have contributed to the creation of this book. In particular, I would like to thank Danielle Graham and Michelle Seo for their translation of the original Korean manuscript into English. Phyllis Elving added an elegant and engaging style to the text with her editing and Mark Rhynsburger polished it with his careful proofreading.

From the beginning, Steve Kim and the staff of Best Life Media tirelessly helped me from the original research and writing, to editing, to the final production. I am grateful for their creativity and professionalism. I also extend great thanks to Jooyoung Ryu, Rebecca Tinkle, and Junghee Lee for the warm illustrations that brought the concepts and methods in this book to life.

Finally, I would like to thank all of the many thousands of individual practitioners who, through their diligence and dedication to their own healing, have helped establish the effectiveness of the Solar Body Method, especially those who were willing to share their personal journey on these pages.

ABOUT THE AUTHOR

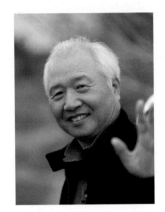

ILCHI LEE is an impassioned visionary, educator, mentor, and innovator; he has dedicated his life to teaching energy principles and researching and developing methods to nurture the full potential of the human brain.

For over thirty years, his life's mission has been to help people harness their own creative power and personal potential. For this goal, he has developed many successful mind-body training methods, including Dahn Yoga and Brain Education. His principles and methods have inspired many people around the world to live healthier and happier lives.

Lee is a *New York Times* bestselling author who has penned thirty-seven books, including *The Call of Sedona: Journey of the Heart*, *Healing Society: A Prescription for Global Enlightenment*, and *Brain Wave Vibration: Getting Back into the Rhythm of a Happy, Healthy Life*.

He is also a well-respected humanitarian who has been working with the United Nations and other organizations for global peace. Lee serves as the president of the University of Brain Education and the International Brain Education Association. For more information about Ilchi Lee and his work, visit ilchi.com

INTERNET RESOURCES

WWW.SOLARBODYMETHOD.COM

The hub of everything for your Solar Body, this site offers support for your practice with up-to-date information about the Solar Body Method and related training techniques for recharging your natural healing power. You'll find:

- full online Solar Body courses.

- quick tips to enhance your practice.

- related products for easy purchase, including Solar Body Circuit Cards and the Solar Body Detox Patch.

- more stories from people who have successfully applied the Solar Body Method to their lives.

- listings for off-line workshops, classes, and retreats.

- related articles about enhancing your natural healing power.

Visit today and gain a wealth of information about the book, the practice, and the author.

SCAN TO WATCH VIDEOS OF SOLAR BODY EXERCISES

INDIVIDUALIZED INSTRUCTION

DAHN YOGA AND BODY & BRAIN CENTERS

Capture the full power of the Solar Body Method with the help of experts. Dahn Yoga and its franchised Body & Brain Centers provide a variety of instructional programs and natural healing workshops based on Ilchi Lee's Solar Body Method. Through classes, workshops, and retreats, perfect your technique and learn the best way to apply the method to your daily life for optimal health.

National leaders in health and wellness, Dahn Yoga Centers and Body & Brain Centers can be found in many major cities around the United States. Their offerings include yoga, tai chi, meditation, and other mind–body training programs based on traditional Korean healing philosophy and East Asian energy principles. Dahn Yoga's holistic methods have been offered in the U.S. through corporate, affiliate, and franchise locations, as well as in community-based classes, for nearly twenty years.

Find the center nearest you at dahnyoga.com.

ONE WEEK FREE CLASSES WITH THIS BOOK

Bring this book to any participating U.S. Dahn Yoga or Body & Brain Center for a free week of unlimited group classes. Offer expires June 30, 2016.

RELATED PRODUCTS

SOLAR ENERGY CIRCUIT CARDS

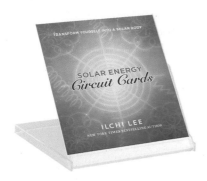

Practice Solar Energy Circuit Training with the help of these 12 colorful meditation cards. Use the cards to remember and visualize the energy circuits described in this book. Easily displayed in their CD case, you can carry the cards with you to connect with the energy circuits you need wherever you are. The cards include a description of each circuit and how to use it to release stagnant energy and power up your natural healing ability. The deck also describes additional Solar Energy Circuit meditation techniques.

SOLAR BODY DETOX PATCH

By stimulating reflexology zones on the soles of your feet, Solar Body Detox Patch is designed to promote the natural detoxification of your body. The foot patch has been used in many Asian countries to combat fatigue, improve circulation, increase metabolism, enhance quality of sleep, help release toxins, and as a general practice to stay healthy and clean. Apply the Solar Body Detox Patch to both feet before bed and let them work while you sleep. See the results in the morning and experience the benefits of cleansing from the inside out!

These products are available at SolarBodyMethod.com.

IMAGE PERMISSIONS ACKNOWLEDGMENTS

Page 18 © Thinkstock.com/kwasny221

Page 49 © Lauri Nummenmaa, Enrico Glerean, Riitta Hari, and Jari Hietanen

Page 58 © Thinkstock.com/Jupiterimages

Page 66 © Thinkstock.com/FotoMaximum

Page 84 © Thinkstock.com/mabe123

Page 142 © Jordan Diamond

Page 164 © Thinkstock.com/yaruta

Page 178 © PeterHermesFurian

Page 184 © Franklin Hughes

Page 208 © Thinkstock.com/OlgaMiltsova

Page 214 © Thinkstock.com/Brand X Pictures

Page 230 © Thinkstock.com/Brand X Pictures